The EBMT/EHA CAR-T Cell Ha

Nicolaus Kröger · John Gribben
Christian Chabannon · Ibrahim Yakoub-Agha
Hermann Einsele
Editors

The EBMT/EHA CAR-T Cell Handbook

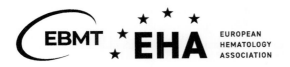

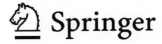

Editors
Nicolaus Kröger (iD)
Department of Stem Cell Transplantation
University Medical Center
Hamburg-Eppendorf
Hamburg, Germany

John Gribben (iD)
Bart's Cancer Institute
Queen Mary University of London
London, UK

Christian Chabannon (iD)
Institut Paoli-Calmettes Comprehensive
Cancer Center
Aix-Marseille Université School of
Medicine
Marseille, France

Ibrahim Yakoub-Agha (iD)
Maladies du Sang
Unité de Thérapie Cellulaire
Centre hospitalier-Universitaire de Lille
Lille, France

Hermann Einsele (iD)
Department of Internal Medicine II
University Hospital Würzburg
Würzburg, Bayern, Germany

ISBN 978-3-030-94352-3   ISBN 978-3-030-94353-0   (eBook)
https://doi.org/10.1007/978-3-030-94353-0

This Springer imprint is published by the registered company Springer Nature Switzerland AG
The registered company address is: Gewerbestrasse 11, 6330 Cham, Switzerland

Preface

Chimeric antigen receptor T cell therapy (CAR-T) is a new class of medicinal products that are genetically engineered from T cells. It is expected that other forms of Immune Effector Cells-based therapies will soon reach the market, manufactured from other subsets of immune cells, and engineered through other technologies than currently used defective retroviral or lentiviral vectors. Cell-based immunotherapies add to the broader field of immunotherapies, now populated with monoclonal antibodies including immune checkpoint inhibitors, immune-conjugates, and bi- and tri-specific antibodies. Approximately 30 years after the first publications reporting on the development of genetically engineered T cells, expression of a first generation chimeric antigen receptor (CAR), and the demonstration of its capability to recognize antigens in the absence of MHC presentation in the 1980s, the first commercially available CAR-T cell medicinal products were approved by the FDA and later by the EMA for the treatment of relapsed/refractory diffuse large B cell lymphoma and relapsed/refractory acute lymphoblastic leukemia.

To foster CAR-T cell development and patients' access to these novel cellular therapies in Europe, the European Society of Blood and Marrow Transplantation (EBMT) and the European Hematology Association (EHA) combined forces from 2018—the year of the first approvals of CAR-T Cells in Europe—by working closely together in the fields of education, scientific developments, and communication with health authority and all other stakeholders. It started with the organization in 2019 of the first and immediately successful edition of an annual and jointly organized European CAR-T cell meeting that has become the premier event in the field on the European continent. Beyond this major educational initiative, the two continental professional associations have established the "GoCART-Coalition" that aims to provide a neutral ecosystem that allows the many interested parties to communicate and commonly search to solve the many hurdles that the field is facing to fully exploit the medical value of these innovative therapies.

In line with this collaboration, the EBMT/EHA Handbook "CAR-T cell therapy"—of which you read the first edition—was developed. The aim of this handbook is to provide the state-of-the-art information on ongoing scientific developments and medical practices in the field of CAR-T cell therapies, to enhance knowledge and practice skills for all categories of healthcare professionals and scientists.

EBMT and EHA want to express their gratitude to the enormous effort of all authors in planning and writing the different chapters and especially Isabel Sánchez-Ortega and Francesco Cerisoli for their continuous and tireless support.

On behalf of EBMT and EHA, we hope this CAR-T cell handbook will be helpful in your daily practice.

Hamburg, Germany	Nicolaus Kröger
London, UK	John Gribben
Marseille, France	Christian Chabannon
Lille, France	Ibrahim Yakoub-Agha
Würzburg, Germany	Hermann Einsele

Contents

Part III Clinical Indications for CAR-T Cells

Part IV Clinical Management of Patients Treated with CAR-T Cells

Part I

The Science Behind CAR-T Cells

Structure of and Signalling Through Chimeric Antigen Receptor

Christian Chabannon ⓘ and Chiara Bonini

Chimeric antigen receptor (CAR) is a synthetic transmembrane protein expressed at the surface of immune effector cells (IECs) that are reprogrammed either in vitro or in vivo (June et al. 2018; June and Sadelain 2018). Techniques for genetic engineering of autologous or allogeneic IECs are described in the next chapter. The synthetic CAR incorporates several functional domains. The extracellular domain is composed of a single chain variable fragment (ScFV) of immunoglobulin and recognizes the "tumour" antigen. The clinical relevance of the selected tumour antigen—with a view to minimize "on-target/off-tumour" side effects—is discussed in the third chapter of this section. Bispecific and trispecific CARs are currently being evaluated in preclinical and early clinical trials (Bielamowicz et al. 2018; Shah et al. 2020). The use of an immunoglobulin domain as the ligand of the target antigen means that recognition is not restricted to HLA antigens and that CAR-T cells are universally applicable as opposed to T cell receptor (TCR) transgenic T cells that recognize antigenic peptides presented in the context of a defined major histocompatibility complex (MHC), limiting clinical applications to subsets of patients with defined HLA typing. The intracellular domain is composed of the intracellular domain of the zeta chain of the CD3 component of the TCR, which will trigger signalling when the CAR engages the targeted ligand. The transmembrane region links the two extracellular and intracellular domains through the cell membrane and plays an important role in determining the conformation and flexibility of the CAR and its ability to efficiently bind the targeted

C. Chabannon (✉)
Institut Paoli-Calmettes, Centre de Lutte Contre le Cancer, Centre d'Investigations Cliniques en Biothérapie, Université d'Aix-Marseille, Inserm CBT-1409, Marseille, France
e-mail: CHABANNONC@ipc.unicancer.fr

C. Bonini
Experimental Hematology Unit, Division of Immunology, Transplantation and Infectious Diseases, Vita-Salute San Raffaele University, IRCCS Ospedale San Raffaele Scientific Institute, Milan, Italy
e-mail: bonini.chiara@hsr.it

© The Author(s) 2022
N. Kröger et al. (eds.), *The EBMT/EHA CAR-T Cell Handbook*,
https://doi.org/10.1007/978-3-030-94353-0_1

antigen/epitope. Association of only these three functional domains characterized first generation CARs, as described in the original publications (Kuwana et al. 1987; Eshhar et al. 1993). However, full activation of T cells requires the addition of one (second generation CARs) or two (third generation CARs) domains from costimulatory molecules, such as CD28, 4-1BB/CD137, or OX40/CD134, that provide the T cell costimulatory signal. Currently approved CAR-T cells are second generation CAR-T cells; as an illustration, the CAR in tisagenlecleucel contains a 4-1BB domain, while the CAR in axicabtagene ciloleucel contains a CD28 domain. The nature of the costimulatory domain influences the ability of CAR-T cells to expand or persist (limit T cell exhaustion) in vivo after infusion into the patient, although it is unclear how this translates clinically and affects disease control, occurrence of adverse events, and overall survival due to the lack of head-to-head comparison between approved products. Finally, fourth generation CAR-T cells have been developed for preclinical projects. These cells, named armoured CAR cells or T cells redirected for universal cytokine-mediated killing (TRUCKS), encode not only a CAR (usually with one costimulatory domain, such as in second generation CARs) but also a cytokine, interleukin, pro-inflammatory ligand, or chemokine that will counteract the immune suppressive microenvironment that prevails in most solid tumours (Eshhar et al. 1993; Chmielewski and Abken 2015).

When the CAR engages its ligand, signalling involves several components of the naturally occurring TCR. These include molecules such as lymphocyte-specific protein tyrosine kinase (LCK). Some components of the signalling cascade are actionable with existing drugs, which offers opportunities for pharmacologic modulation of CAR activity in vivo, such as described with tyrosine kinase inhibitors (Mestermann et al. 2019; Weber et al. 2019); this represents an appealing alternative to the inclusion of a suicide gene in the CAR construct (Casucci et al. 2013; Gargett and Brown 2014; Sakemura et al. 2016). Synthetic biology applied to the CAR-T cell field led to engineering of combinatorial antigen recognition constructs. The "OR" gate strategy (i.e., CD19 and CD22) allows CAR-T cell activation upon recognition of at least 1 of the 2 targeted antigens, thus reducing the risk of cancer immune evasion. The "OR" and "NOT" gate strategies are designed to improve the safety profile of CAR-T cells, since tumour cells and healthy cells can be discriminated by CAR-T cells based on the expression pattern of 2 antigens (Weber et al. 2020).

Key Points
- A chimeric antigen receptor is a synthetic transmembrane molecule encoded by a DNA sequence that combines domains from immunoglobulins, one chain of the T cell receptor, and typically domains from costimulatory molecules involved in T cell activation.
- Currently approved and commercially available CAR-T cells are second generation CAR-T cells that contain a single costimulatory domain.
- The machinery for cell signalling contains actionable elements, thus offering opportunities for in vivo modulation of CAR-T cell activities and mitigation of adverse events.

References

Bielamowicz K, Fousek K, Byrd TT, Samaha H, Mukherjee M, Aware N, et al. Trivalent CAR-T cells overcome interpatient antigenic variability in glioblastoma. Neuro-Oncology. 2018;20(4):506–18.

Casucci M, Nicolis di Robilant B, Falcone L, Camisa B, Norelli M, Genovese P, et al. CD44v6-targeted T cells mediate potent antitumor effects against acute myeloid leukemia and multiple myeloma. Blood. 2013;122(20):3461–72.

Chmielewski M, Abken H. TRUCKs: the fourth generation of CARs. Expert Opin Biol Ther. 2015;15(8):1145–54.

Eshhar Z, Waks T, Gross G, Schindler DG. Specific activation and targeting of cytotoxic lymphocytes through chimeric single chains consisting of antibody-binding domains and the gamma or zeta subunits of the immunoglobulin and T-cell receptors. Proc Natl Acad Sci U S A. 1993;90(2):720–4.

Gargett T, Brown MP. The inducible caspase-9 suicide gene system as a "safety switch" to limit on-target, off-tumor toxicities of chimeric antigen receptor T cells. Front Pharmacol. 2014;5:235.

June CH, Sadelain M. Chimeric antigen receptor therapy. N Engl J Med. 2018;379(1):64–73.

June CH, O'Connor RS, Kawalekar OU, Ghassemi S, Milone MC. CAR-T cell immunotherapy for human cancer. Science. 2018;359(6382):1361–5.

Kuwana Y, Asakura Y, Utsunomiya N, Nakanishi M, Arata Y, Itoh S, et al. Expression of chimeric receptor composed of immunoglobulin-derived V regions and T-cell receptor-derived C regions. Biochem Biophys Res Commun. 1987;149(3):960–8.

Mestermann K, Giavridis T, Weber J, Rydzek J, Frenz S, Nerreter T, et al. The tyrosine kinase inhibitor dasatinib acts as a pharmacologic on/off switch for CAR-T cells. Sci Transl Med. 2019;11(499):eaau5907.

Sakemura R, Terakura S, Watanabe K, Julamanee J, Takagi E, Miyao K, et al. A Tet-On inducible system for controlling CD19-chimeric antigen receptor expression upon drug administration. Cancer Immunol Res. 2016;4(8):658–68.

Shah NN, Johnson BD, Schneider D, Zhu F, Szabo A, Keever-Taylor CA, et al. Bispecific anti-CD20, anti-CD19 CAR-T cells for relapsed B cell malignancies: a phase 1 dose escalation and expansion trial. Nat Med. 2020;26(10):1569–75.

Weber EW, Lynn RC, Sotillo E, Lattin J, Xu P, Mackall CL. Pharmacologic control of CAR-T cell function using dasatinib. Blood Adv. 2019;3(5):711–7.

Weber EW, Maus MV, Mackall CL. The emerging landscape of immune cell therapies. Cell. 2020;181(1):46–62.

Genetic Engineering of Autologous or Allogeneic Immune Effector Cells

Karim Benabdellah, Simone Thomas, and Hinrich Abken

Manufacturing immune effector cells (T or NK cells) with CAR-encoding DNA sequences requires efficient and safe genetic engineering procedures. For this purpose, an appropriate genetic vector is chosen according to numerous factors, including the vector genome packaging capacity, cellular tropism, genomic integration, immune toxicity, and other factors. In clinical trials, genomes integrating viral vectors, in particular vectors based on members of the *Retroviridae* family, such as retroviruses and lentiviruses, have been successfully used for more than 20 years. These vectors contain an RNA genome that when transcribed into double-stranded DNA by reverse transcriptase integrates into the genome of the transduced cell.

Several precautions are taken to ensure the safe use of such integrating vectors. First, the viral genome is split into three different expression constructs to reduce the risk of recombination events re-establishing replication-competent viruses. Second, long terminal repeats (LTRs) with their enhancer/promoter sequences are deleted, resulting in self-inactivated (SIN) vectors to avoid transactivation of cellular genes in the vicinity of the viral integration site. Third, the viral envelope is pseudotyped with heterologous glycoproteins, such as gibbon ape leukaemia virus

K. Benabdellah
Centre for Genomics and Oncological Research (GENYO), Genomic Medicine Department, Pfizer-University of Granada-Andalusian Regional Government, Granada, Spain
e-mail: karim.benabdel@genyo.es

S. Thomas
Department of Genetic Immunotherapy, Regensburg Center for Interventional Immunology, Regensburg, Germany

Department of Internal Medicine III, University Hospital Regensburg, Regensburg, Germany
e-mail: Simone.Thomas@klinik.uni-regensburg.de

H. Abken (✉)
Department of Genetic Immunotherapy, Regensburg Center for Interventional Immunology, Regensburg, Germany
e-mail: hinrich.abken@ukr.de

© The Author(s) 2022
N. Kröger et al. (eds.), *The EBMT/EHA CAR-T Cell Handbook*,
https://doi.org/10.1007/978-3-030-94353-0_2

(GALV) or vesicular stomatitis virus (VSV)-G protein, to restrict the cell tropism for transduction. The viral vectors have undergone generations of modifications and are classified according to their packaging plasmid. During manufacturing, the use of transduction enhancers, including cationic polymers, lipids, and peptides, such as Retronectin or Vectofusin-1, which is a histidine-rich cationic amphipathic short peptide (Jamali et al. 2019), improves the transduction efficiencies.

Retroviral vectors modified with the LTRs of the myeloproliferative sarcoma virus and an improved 5′ untranslated region, named MP71 retroviral vectors, can achieve high transduction efficiencies in human T cells. While retroviral vectors require actively dividing cells for integration, lentiviral vectors have the capacity to transduce nondividing or slowly proliferating cells and are currently increasingly used for genetic modification of T cells in clinical trials. Cycling T cells can efficiently complete the reverse transcription process of the viral vector, facilitate nuclear import, and enhance the expression of the transgene. Obtaining high virus titres and ultimately sufficient transduction frequencies for production of CAR-T cells on a clinical scale and preserving the T cell phenotype and functional properties after transduction remain a challenge. Despite vector integration into the host genome, T cells have a negligible risk of transformation; thus far, no leukaemia has been observed in T cell-based therapy.

Alternatively, artificial virus-like particles (VLPs) pseudotyped with VSV-G can be used for transfer into haematopoietic cells (Mangeot et al. 2019). DNA packed into transposon vectors, such as sleeping beauty and piggyBac, are transferred to T cells via electroporation (Kebriaei et al. 2016). Transposon-based genetic engineering does not require time-consuming and cost-intensive virus production and is increasingly considered for clinical manufacture of CAR-T cells.

In contrast to integrating DNA transfer technologies, mRNA transfer via electroporation or cationic lipid-mediated transfection produces T cells with transient CAR expression for a few days (Miliotou and Papadopoulou 2020). Such transient CAR-T cell approaches have been investigated and found to produce antitumour reactivity for a limited time to avoid any undesirable effects in patients; however, very few clinical trials using RNA-modified CAR-T cells have been registered.

Genome editing is an upcoming tool to engineer CAR-T cells using specific endonucleases, including meganucleases (MGNs), transcription activator-like effector nucleases (TALENs), megaTAL nucleases, zinc-finger nucleases (ZFNs) and, more recently, clustered regularly interspaced short palindromic repeat (CRISPR)-Cas9-associated nucleases (Pavlovic et al. 2020). These technologies allow insertion of a specific DNA sequence at a predefined emplacement, such as endogenous genetic locus. While efficiently applied in haematopoietic or mesenchymal stem cell modification for years, genome editing in primary T cells has only recently been successfully applied towards efficient CAR-T cell engineering. Examples for potential clinical application are targeting the respective genes for programmed cell death-1 (PD1, CD279), T cell receptor (TCR) α and β chains, CD52, human leukocyte antigens (HLAs), and β2-microglobulin (β2M).

One major application of genome editing is creating "off-the-shelf" alloge-neic CAR-T cells to avoid certain limitations associated with autologous T cells, such as the personalized production process, the several weeks of time required for manufacturing, and the risk of manufacturing failure. Such allogeneic CAR-T cells were engineered by genetically eliminating the TCRα constant (TRAC) locus and/or HLA from the T cell surface, reducing the risk of graft versus host disease (GvHD) and allograft rejection. In particular, Torikai et al. combined sleeping beauty transposon-based gene transfer with ZFN-mediated deletion of TCR α and β chains (Torikai et al. 2012); subsequent approaches also eliminated the endogenous TCR (Roth et al. 2018; Legut et al. 2018; Osborn et al. 2016). TALEN-mediated TRAC/CD52 knockout of CD19-specific CAR-T cells (UCART19) was administered to two patients with relapsed ALL in a proof-of-concept study, and no GvHD was reported (Qasim et al. 2017). Several approaches using ZFNs and CRISPR/Cas9, including base editing variants, were used to eliminate HLA class I expression by targeting β2M (Webber et al. 2019) and eliminating the HLA class II transactivator CIITA (Kagoya et al. 2020), all reducing the risk of allogeneic CAR-T cell rejection. To reduce GvHD and fratricide, the CD7 locus was disrupted along with TCRα editing (Gomes-Silva et al. 2017). Eliminating the gene for the TGF-β receptor or PD-1 enhanced CAR-T cell antitumour potency by reducing repression by the tumour stroma (Tang et al. 2020).

Genome editing has also been used to insert the CAR-encoding DNA sequence into the TCR α locus (Eyquem et al. 2017), thereby utilizing the TCR expression machinery for properly regulated CAR expression. Similarly, CAR-encoding DNA was inserted into the TCR α locus, and IL-12-encoding DNA was inserted into the IL2Rα or PDCD1 locus, resulting in CAR-redirected T cell activation along with IL-12 secretion (Sachdeva et al. 2019). Such genome editing approaches can be applied to target other signalling pathways to engineer CAR-T cells with therapeutic outputs in a highly regulated manner. Currently, most of these editing technologies are being explored in mouse models or in a very limited number of patients, making it difficult to draw a definitive conclusion concerning safety and efficacy in the long term.

Key Points
- Lentiviral gene transfer is the most frequently applied procedure to engineer CAR-T cells for clinical use.
- Nonviral transposon-mediated DNA transfer is an upcoming technology to obtain CAR-T cells.
- Allogeneic "off-the-shelf" CAR-T cells are engineered by genetically eliminating the TCRα constant (TRAC) locus and/or HLA from the T cell surface, reducing the risk of graft versus host disease (GvHD) and allograft rejection.

References

Eyquem J, Mansilla-Soto J, Giavridis T, et al. Targeting a CAR-T o the TRAC locus with CRISPR/Cas9 enhances tumour rejection. Nature. 2017;543:113–7.

Gomes-Silva D, Srinivasan M, Sharma S, et al. CD7-edited T cells expressing a CD7-specific CAR for the therapy of T-cell malignancies. Blood. 2017;130:285–96.

Jamali A, Kapitza L, Schaser T, et al. Highly efficient and selective CAR-gene transfer using CD4- and CD8-targeted lentiviral vectors. Mol Ther Methods Clin Dev. 2019;13:371–9.

Kagoya Y, Guo T, Yeung B, et al. Genetic ablation of HLA class I, class II, and the T-cell receptor enables allogeneic T cells to be used for adoptive T-cell therapy. Cancer Immunol Res. 2020;8:926–36.

Kebriaei P, Singh H, Huls MH, et al. Phase I trials using sleeping beauty to generate CD19-specific CAR-T cells. J Clin Invest. 2016;126:3363–76.

Legut M, Dolton G, Mian AA, et al. CRISPR-mediated TCR replacement generates superior anti-cancer transgenic T cells. Blood. 2018;131:311–22.

Mangeot PE, Risson V, Fusil F, et al. Genome editing in primary cells and in vivo using viral-derived nanoblades loaded with Cas9-sgRNA ribonucleoproteins. Nat Commun. 2019;10:45.

Miliotou AN, Papadopoulou LC. In vitro-transcribed (IVT)-mRNA CAR-T therapy development. Methods Mol Biol. 2020;2086:87–117.

Osborn MJ, Webber BR, Knipping F, et al. Evaluation of TCR gene editing achieved by TALENs, CRISPR/Cas9, and megaTAL nucleases. Mol Ther. 2016;24:570–81.

Pavlovic K, Tristán-Manzano M, Maldonado-Pérez N, et al. Using gene editing approaches to fine-tune the immune system. Front Immunol. 2020;11:570672.

Qasim W, Zhan H, Samarasinghe S, et al. Molecular remission of infant B-ALL after infusion of universal TALEN gene-edited CAR-T cells. Sci Transl Med. 2017;9:eaaj2013.

Roth TL, Puig-Saus C, Yu R, et al. Reprogramming human T cell function and specificity with non-viral genome targeting. Nature. 2018;559:405–9.

Sachdeva M, Busser BW, Temburni S, et al. Repurposing endogenous immune pathways to tailor and control chimeric antigen receptor T cell functionality. Nat Commun. 2019;10:5100.

Tang N, Cheng C, Zhang X, et al. TGF-beta inhibition via CRISPR promotes the long-term efficacy of CAR-T cells against solid tumors. JCI Insight. 2020;5:e133977.

Torikai H, Reik A, Liu PQ, et al. A foundation for universal T-cell based immunotherapy: T cells engineered to express a CD19-specific chimeric-antigen-receptor and eliminate expression of endogenous TCR. Blood. 2012;119:5697–705.

Webber BR, Lonetree CL, Kluesner MG, et al. Highly efficient multiplex human T cell engineering without double-strand breaks using Cas9 base editors. Nat Commun. 2019;10:5222.

What Defines a Good Tumour Antigen?

Emma C. Morris and J. H. F. (Fred) Falkenburg

Compared to standard anticancer therapies, such as chemotherapy, small molecule inhibitors and radiation, T cell immunotherapies have the advantages of a high degree of specificity and durability of response typically associated with cellular therapies. The functional specificity of a T cell is determined by its antigen recognition receptor and the target antigen (Bjorkman et al. 1987; Garcia et al. 1996).

The majority of CAR-T cells currently applied in clinical practice do not recognize tumour-specific target antigens but pan-B cell antigens (CD19, CD20, CD22) or maturation antigens (e.g., BCMA), which are abundantly expressed cell surface molecules on both malignant and normal cells (Sadelain et al. 2017; June and Sadelain 2018). In reality, these are only 'ideal' or 'good' tumour antigens because the depletion of normal B cells is generally well tolerated. In contrast to endogenous T cell receptors (TCRs), which are HLA-restricted and recognize peptide-MHC complexes on the target cell surface, CARs recognize extracellular, membrane-bound targets. These are typically nonpolymorphic proteins or glycoproteins. This is advantageous over TCR-mediated recognition because CAR-T cell therapies are not limited by patient HLA type.

What defines a 'good' tumour antigen for recognition by a CAR-T cell?

1. Extracellular expression (i.e., expressed on the cell surface and readily accessible)
2. Uniform or consistent expression on all malignant cells
3. Not subject to downregulation or deletion (i.e., no escape variants). This only occurs if the antigen is a molecule critical for maintenance of the malignant population

E. C. Morris (✉)
Institute of Immunity and Transplantation, University College London, London, UK
e-mail: e.morris@ucl.ac.uk

J. H. F. (Fred) Falkenburg
Leiden University Medical Center, Leiden, The Netherlands
e-mail: j.h.falkenburg@lumc.nl

N. Kröger et al. (eds.), *The EBMT/EHA CAR-T Cell Handbook*,
https://doi.org/10.1007/978-3-030-94353-0_3

4. Should be expressed on malignant stem cells, and
5. Should not be expressed on normal tissue cells, at least not in nonessential normal tissues (i.e., tumour specific).

Tumour-Specific Antigens (TSAs)

TSAs are highly specific and typically result from genetic mutations within malignant cells that give rise to neoantigens not present in untransformed (nonmalignant) cells (Schumacher and Schreiber 2015; Schumacher et al. 2019). By definition, there is a low likelihood of 'on-target off-tumour' toxicity because the tumour antigen is not expressed on normal cells. 'On-target on-tumour' toxicities and 'off-target off-tumour' toxicities may occur as a result of CRS or receptor cross-reactivity. Unfortunately, no nonpolymorphic tumour-specific extracellular target antigens are known. The only highly specific extracellular tumour target antigens are neopeptides presented in the context of (polymorphic) HLA molecules.

Multiple Tumour Antigens Resulting in a 'Tumour-Specific Phenotype'

Recent studies have demonstrated that simultaneous targeting of two or more target antigens may improve tumour specificity and reduce the risk of antigen escape (Shah et al. 2020; Dai et al. 2020). In such cases, one target antigen may be lineage-specific but not tumour specific, but the combination may be tumour specific. For CAR-T cells to be fully activated, the target cell must express both target antigens (i.e., combined antigen expression). This approach is not expected to ameliorate the risk of CRS, and it is difficult to estimate the risk of 'on-target off-tumour' toxicity, which will depend on the ability of CAR-T cells to discriminate between cells with combined or single antigen expression. In this case, there would be a potential risk of 'off-target off-tumour' toxicity for single antigens (expression of a single antigen in normal cells or aberrant antigen expression in normal cells).

Lineage-Specific and Differentiation Antigens

These antigens are commonly targeted by CAR-T cells and include CD19, CD20, CD22, and BCMA, which are B cell lineage antigens. Lineage-specific antigens can be optimal targets in the case of tumours associated with cell lineages and/or tissues that are nonredundant or temporarily replaceable, such as the B cell lineage, plasma cells, and thyroid, prostate, and ovarian cells. In these circumstances, their function can be rescued by a second therapeutic intervention. For example, profound B cell lymphopenia following CD19 CAR-T cell therapy can result in hypogammaglobulinaemia and absent or impaired vaccine responses, requiring long-term immunoglobulin replacement therapy. More recent developments aimed at generating

CAR-T cells for treatment of AML and other myeloid malignancies target lineage-specific and differentiation antigens (i.e., CD33 and CD123) but risk profound cytopenia or bone marrow aplasia and depend on the ability to subsequently replace haematopoietic stem cells and myeloid precursors (Gill et al. 2014). Recent preclinical studies have attempted to fine-tune CAR-T cell responses through the incorporation of safety switch mechanisms (Loff et al. 2020). In the case of lineage-specific antigens, 'on-target off-tumour' toxicity is common, resulting in depletion of specific cell lineages or other cells in the case of aberrant antigen expression. CRS may be common, due in part to wide antigen expression in both normal and malignant cells.

Lineage-Specific Polymorphic/Heterogeneic Antigens

These target antigens are similar to lineage-specific antigens (above) with the advantage that only part of the system is eliminated (following CAR-T cell targeting) due to intrinsic heterogeneity or antigen expression. Examples include targeting immunoglobulin subclasses or kappa versus lambda light chains in association with immunoglobulin receptors.

Key Points
1. Most CAR-T cells and all currently approved products target lineage-specific antigens.
2. This results in loss of nonmalignant cells that also express these antigens (e.g., normal B cells).
3. With commercially available CAR-T products, these side effects are manageable but may be more limiting with other novel targets under development.

References

Bjorkman PJ, Saper MA, Samraoui B, et al. Structure of the human class I histocompatibility antigen, HLA-A2. Nature. 1987;329(6139):506–12.
Dai H, Wu Z, Jia H, et al. Bispecific CAR-T cells targeting both CD19 and CD22 for therapy of adults with relapsed or refractory B cell acute lymphoblastic leukemia. J Hematol Oncol. 2020;13(1):30.
Garcia KC, Degano M, Stanfield RL, et al. An alphabeta T cell receptor structure at 2.5 A and its orientation in the TCR-MHC complex. Science. 1996;274(5285):209–19.
Gill S, Tasian SK, Ruella M, et al. Preclinical targeting of human acute myeloid leukemia and myeloablation using chimeric antigen receptor-modified T cells. Blood. 2014;123:2343–54.
June CH, Sadelain M. Chimeric antigen receptor therapy. N Engl J Med. 2018;379:64–73.
Loff S, Dietrich J, Meyer JE, et al. Rapidly switchable universal CAR-T cells for treatment of CD123-positive leukemia. Mol Ther Oncolytics. 2020;17:408–20.
Sadelain M, Rivière I, Riddell S. Therapeutic T cell engineering. Nature. 2017;545:423–31.

Schumacher TN, Schreiber RD. Neoantigens in cancer immunotherapy. Science. 2015;348:69–74.

Schumacher TN, Scheper W, Kvistborg P. Annu Rev Immunol. 2019;37:172–200.

Shah NN, Johnson BD, Schneider D, et al. Bispecific anti-CD20, anti-CD19 CAR-T cells for relapsed B cell malignancies: a phase 1 dose escalation and expansion trial. Nat Med. 2020;26(10):1569–75.

Tumour Escape from CAR-T Cells

4

Leo Rasche, Luca Vago, and Tuna Mutis

Over the past decade, CAR-T cells have emerged as one of the most powerful cellular immune therapy approaches in the battle against haematological malignancies. Nonetheless, similar to other immunotherapeutic approaches, tumour cells develop strategies to evade CAR-T cell therapy, often with the support of a highly immunosuppressive and protective tumour microenvironment. To date, antigen loss, immune dysfunction, exhaustion and (microenvironment-mediated) upregulation of anti-apoptotic pathways have been identified as major modes of tumour escape from CAR-T cell therapy. This chapter will focus on our current understanding of these modes of immune escape from CAR-T cells.

Leo Rasche, Luca Vago and Tuna Mutis contributed equally with all other contributors.

L. Rasche
Department of Internal Medicine 2, University Hospital of Würzburg, Würzburg, Germany

Mildred Scheel Early Career Center, University Hospital of Würzburg, Würzburg, Germany
e-mail: rasche_l@ukw.de

L. Vago
Vita-Salute San Raffaele University, Milan, Italy

Unit of Immunogenetics, Leukemia Genomics and Immunobiology, IRCCS San Raffaele
Scientific Institute, Milan, Italy
e-mail: vago.luca@hsr.it

T. Mutis (✉)
Department of Hematology, Amsterdam University Medical Centers, Location VUmc,
Amsterdam, The Netherlands
e-mail: t.mutis@amsterdamumc.nl

© The Author(s) 2022
N. Kröger et al. (eds.), *The EBMT/EHA CAR-T Cell Handbook*,
https://doi.org/10.1007/978-3-030-94353-0_4

15

Immune Escape and CAR-T Cell Resistance Related to Antigen Loss

Antigen loss represents the ultimate adaptation of a cancer cell to the selective pressure of targeted immunotherapy. While antigen downregulation or dim expression is a well-known event in lymphoma and myeloma treated with therapeutic IgG antibodies (Plesner et al. 2020; Jilani et al. 2003), complete target loss is a phenomenon typically occurring after T-cell-based therapy, such as CAR-T cell or T cell engaging bispecific antibodies (TCE) therapy, and rarely after treatment with antibody-drug conjugates (ADCs).

In B cell malignancies, CD19 loss has been noted in up to 40% of patients with B cell acute lymphoblastic leukaemia treated with different CAR 19 products (Orlando et al. 2018). Point mutations in CD19 have been described to lead to nonfunctional anchoring of the CD19 protein to the cell membrane and consequently to a loss of surface antigen (Orlando et al. 2018). Deleterious mutations and alternatively spliced CD19 mRNA variants were identified in two other studies (Asnani et al. 2020; Sotillo et al. 2015). In B-ALL with rearrangement of the mixed lineage leukaemia (MLL) gene, some patients relapsed with clonally related acute myeloid leukaemia after treatment with CD19 CAR-T cells, adding a switch to a CD19-negative myeloid phenotype as another mechanism of resistance (Gardner et al. 2016). In DLBCL, the frequency of CD19 loss after CAR19 axicabtagene ciloleucel (axi-cel) treatment was 33% (Neelapu et al. 2017; Neelapu et al. 2019), and alternatively spliced CD19 mRNA species could be identified. In follicular lymphoma and DLBCL treated with CD20 X CD3 bispecific TCE, CD20 loss relapses were seen, but the frequency is yet to be reported (Bannerji et al. 2018). Furthermore, a single case of CD22 loss was described after ADC inotuzumab-ozogamicin treatment in a paediatric patient with B-ALL (Paul et al. 2019). Taken together, antigen loss is a key mechanism of resistance to novel immunotherapies targeting CD19, CD20, and CD22. In myeloma, downregulation of BCMA was recorded in a significant proportion of patients following BCMA CAR-T therapy, but intensity increased back towards baseline in almost all patients (Cohen et al. 2019). However, three case reports described irreversible BCMA loss after anti-BCMA CAR-T cell treatment (Da Via et al. 2021; Samur et al. 2020; Leblay et al. 2020). In two of these cases, homozygous *BCMA* gene deletions were identified as the biological underpinning of antigen loss. In the third case, the authors found a heterozygous *BCMA* deletion together with a *BCMA* mutation, leading to antigen loss. In summary, biallelic events impacting the *BCMA* locus represent one molecular mechanism of antigen loss after BCMA CAR-T therapy. However, these events seem to be rare. In the KarMMa trial, only 4% of patients relapsed without an increase in soluble BCMA, which is thought to be a biomarker of this type of resistance (Munshi et al. 2021). Heterozygous BCMA deletions, present in approximately 7% of anti-BCMA naïve patients, represent a risk factor for BCMA loss-relapse after T-cell-based therapy (Da Via et al. 2021). While a plethora of alternative antigens, such as FCRH5 or GPRC5D, are currently being investigated in early clinical trials (Rasche et al. 2020), antigen loss for these targets has not been reported thus far. However, MM is a disease associated with high frequencies of copy number aberrations, including deletions impacting genes encoding immunotherapy targets, and we expect biallelic events leading to antigen loss to also be relevant for MM targets other than BCMA. Multispecific CAR-T cells or combinations of monospecific targeted immunotherapies may overcome antigen loss in future trials (Fernández de Larrea et al. 2020).

Immune Dysfunction and Exhaustion of CAR-T Cells

In addition to antigen loss, a number of other mechanisms also limit or abrogate the effective recognition of cancer cells by CAR-T cells, either directly conveyed by tumour cells or through rewiring of the microenvironment. In preclinical models, especially in solid tumours, it was shown that tumour-infiltrating CAR-T cells undergo rapid loss of functionality, limiting their therapeutic efficacy. This hyporesponsiveness appears to be reversible when the T cells are isolated away from the tumour and is associated with upregulation of intrinsic T cell inhibitory enzymes (diacylglycerol kinase and SHP-1) and with the expression of surface inhibitory receptors (PD1, LAG3, TIM3, and 2B4) (Moon et al. 2014).

Additionally, in patients with diffuse large B cell lymphoma (DLBCL) treated with axicabtagene ciloleucel (axi-cel), it has been shown that tumour-infiltrating CAR-T cells express the inhibitory receptor PD1 and that they represent only a minor fraction of the immune cells detectable in the tumour (Chen et al. 2020). Of note, immunogenic chemotherapy can enhance the recruitment of CAR-T cells to the tumour bed by inducing the release of chemokines from monocytes, and this can potently synergize with immune checkpoint blockade (Srivastava et al. 2021). In another recent study in DLCBL, interferon (IFN) signalling expression, along with high blood levels of monocytic myeloid-derived suppressor cells (M-MDSCs), IL-6 and ferritin, was associated with a lack of a durable response to axi-cel. The authors showed that high IFN signalling is associated with the expression of multiple checkpoint ligands, including PD-L1, on lymphoma cells and that these levels were higher in patients who lacked a durable response to CAR-T therapy (Jain et al. 2021). However, impairment of IFN signalling, such as through mutations or downmodulation of JAK2 and other pathway components, can confer tumour cell resistance to killing by CAR-redirected T cells (Arenas et al. 2021).

These findings have direct implications for the design of next-generation CAR-T cell protocols: a number of strategies are now being explored to combine immune checkpoint blockade with CAR-T cell therapy, either by coinfusion of genetically modified lymphocytes with monoclonal antibodies or by engineering the cell to produce the relevant scFv (Carneiro and El-Deiry 2020), be resistant to inhibitory signals (Cullen et al. 2010), or even transform signals under activating stimuli (Sutton et al. 2000). Moreover, novel promising compounds have been shown to counteract the activity of T cell inhibitory enzymes (Moon et al. 2014).

Microenvironment-Mediated Tumour Resistance to CAR-T Cells

Immune suppression or exhaustion is not the only mechanism by which tumour cells can become less susceptible to CAR-T cell-mediated cytotoxicity. In many haematological cancers, the bone marrow tumour microenvironment (BMME) is known to upregulate antiapoptotic mechanisms in tumour cells through tight cross-talk of mesenchymal stromal cells (MSCs) and tumour cells. Remarkably, tumour cell lysis by T and NK cells is also largely mediated via activation of extrinsic and intrinsic apoptosis pathways (Hanabuchi et al. 1994; Falschlehner et al. 2009; Carneiro and El-Deiry 2020; Cullen et al. 2010; Sutton et al. 2000). Thus, the idea that BMMSCs might also induce resistance to T and MK cell-mediated cytotoxic activity through upregulation of antiapoptotic mechanisms has recently been tested, and the results showed that MM cell-BMMSC interactions can indeed protect MM cells from conventional cytotoxic T cells and from (daratumumab redirected) NK cells (McMillin et al. 2012; de Haart et al. 2013; de Haart et al. 2016). These studies were recently extended to CAR-T cells by testing a panel of nine different MM-reactive CAR-T cells that were reactive to three different MM-associated antigens (CD138, BCMA, and CD38) with different target affinities and with different costimulatory domains (CD28, 4-1BB, or CD28 plus 4-1BB) (Holthof et al. 2021a). In the absence of BMMSCs, BCMA[bb2121] CAR-T cells, high affinity CD38 CAR-T cells, and intermediate affinity CD38 CAR-T cells containing CD28 costimulatory domains showed high levels of anti-MM cell lysis, whereas other CAR-T cells showed moderate cytotoxic activity against MM cells. BMMSCs did not modulate the lytic activity of highly lytic CAR-T cells but readily protected MM cells against all other CAR-T cells with intermediate killing capacity. Overall, a strong inverse correlation was demonstrated between the lytic capacity of the CAR-T cells and the extent of BMMSC-mediated protection. Furthermore, the BMMSC-mediated protection of MM cells from these CAR-T cells was readily abrogated by inhibition of survivin, MCL-1, and Xiap using the small molecule FL118. Thus, the results confirmed that BMMSC-mediated immune resistance was mediated by negative regulation of apoptotic pathways. In addition, the importance of the tumour stroma in the efficacy of CAR-T cells has also been suggested in a solid tumour mouse model, where destruction of the tumour stroma contributed to eradication of large tumours by HER2-specific CAR-T cells (Textor et al. 2014). Based on these studies, overcoming BMMSC-mediated immune resistance seems possible by increasing the overall avidity and killing activity of CAR-T cells. This may be achieved by designing CARs containing high affinity antigen recognition domains, tandem CARs, or dual CAR strategies (van der Schans et al. 2020). Alternatively, using the CD28 costimulatory domain (Drent et al. 2019; Drent et al. 2017) or engineering CAR-T cells with cytotoxic effector molecules can upregulate CAR-T cell activity. Indeed, it has recently been demonstrated that BMSMSC-mediated immune resistance towards the NK cell line KHYG-1 can be abrogated by engineering it with a CD38 CAR and/or with a DR5-specific, optimized TRAIL variant (Holthof et al. 2021b). CAR-T cells may also be equipped with caspase-independent apoptotic molecules, such as granzyme-A (Borner and Monney 1999).

In addition, a number of earlier and recent studies indicate the importance of apoptotic pathways for the efficacy of other CAR-T cells. For instance, CD19 CAR-T cells were previously found to benefit from combination with the BCL-2 inhibitor ABT-737 (Karlsson et al. 2013). Recently, similar results were observed when third-generation CD19 CAR-T cells were combined with another BCL-2 inhibitor, ABT199 (Yang et al. 2019). Finally, two independent loss-of-function screens in ALL cell lines identified impaired death receptor pathways as another mechanism of resistance to CD19-targeted CAR therapy. Loss of FADD, BID, and tumour necrosis factor-related apoptosis-inducing ligand 2 (TRAIL2) in leukaemia cells was shown to render them more resistant to cytotoxicity and to drive T cell exhaustion upon prolonged stimulation (Singh et al. 2020; Dufva et al. 2020). The combination of CAR-T cells with the SMAC mimetic compound birinapant significantly improved the lysis of malignant cells (Dufva et al. 2020). Thus, when increasing the lytic capacity of CAR-T cells is not possible or desirable, especially if the target antigen is not entirely tumour-specific, tumour cells can be made more sensitive by combining CAR-T cells with small molecules targeting regulatory proteins in the intrinsic and extrinsic apoptotic pathways, as shown in these studies.

Key Points
1. Loss of expression of the target antigen on tumour cells via the selective immune pressure of CAR-T cells is a major mechanism of CAR-T cell therapy failure.
2. T cell exhaustion of CAR-T cells can decrease their function.
3. Multiple other cells in the tumour microenvironment can contribute to inhibition of CAR-T cell function.

References

Arenas EJ, Martínez-Sabadell A, Rius Ruiz I, Román Alonso M, Escorihuela M, Luque A, et al. Acquired cancer cell resistance to T cell bispecific antibodies and CAR-T targeting HER2 through JAK2 down-modulation. Nature. Communications. 2021;12(1):1237.

Asnani M, Hayer KE, Naqvi AS, Zheng S, Yang SY, Oldridge D, et al. Retention of CD19 intron 2 contributes to CART-19 resistance in leukemias with subclonal frameshift mutations in CD19. Leukemia. 2020;34:1202–7.

Bannerji R, Arnason JE, Advani R, Brown JR, Allan JN, Ansell SM, et al. Emerging clinical activity of REGN1979, an anti-CD20 x anti-CD3 bispecific antibody, in patients with relapsed/ refractory follicular lymphoma (FL), diffuse large B-cell lymphoma (DLBCL), and other B-cell non-Hodgkin lymphoma (B-NHL) subtypes. Blood. 2018;132(Suppl 1):1690.

Borner C, Monney L. Apoptosis without caspases: an inefficient molecular guillotine? Cell Death Differ. 1999;6(6):497–507.

Carneiro BA, El-Deiry WS. Targeting apoptosis in cancer therapy. Nat Rev Clin Oncol. 2020;17(7):395–417.

Chen P-H, Lipschitz M, Weirather JL, Jacobson C, Armand P, Wright K, et al. Activation of CAR and non-CAR-T cells within the tumor microenvironment following CAR-T cell therapy. JCI Insight. 2020;5(12):e134612.

Cohen AD, Garfall AL, Stadtmauer EA, Melenhorst JJ, Lacey SF, Lancaster E, et al. B cell maturation antigen-specific CAR-T cells are clinically active in multiple myeloma. J Clin Invest. 2019;129(6):2210–21.

Cullen SP, Brunet M, Martin SJ. Granzymes in cancer and immunity. Cell Death Differ. 2010;17(4):616–23.

Da Via MC, Dietrich O, Truger M, Arampatzi P, Duell J, Heidemeier A, et al. Homozygous BCMA gene deletion in response to anti-BCMA CAR-T cells in a patient with multiple myeloma. Nat Med. 2021;27:616–9.

Drent E, Themeli M, Poels R, de Jong-Korlaar R, Yuan H, de Bruijn J, et al. A rational strategy for reducing on-target off-tumor effects of CD38-chimeric antigen receptors by affinity optimization. Mol Ther. 2017;25(8):1946–58.

Drent E, Poels R, Ruiter R, van de Donk N, Zweegman S, Yuan H, et al. Combined CD28 and 4-1BB costimulation potentiates affinity-tuned chimeric antigen receptor-engineered T cells. Clin Cancer Res. 2019;25(13):4014–25.

Dufva O, Koski J, Maliniemi P, Ianevski A, Klievink J, Leitner J, et al. Integrated drug profiling and CRISPR screening identify essential pathways for CAR-T cell cytotoxicity. Blood. 2020;135(9):597–609.

Falschlehner C, Schaefer U, Walczak H. Following TRAIL's path in the immune system. Immunology. 2009;127(2):145–54.

Fernández de Larrea C, Staehr M, Lopez AV, Ng KY, Chen Y, Godfrey WD, et al. Defining an optimal dual-targeted CAR-T cell therapy approach simultaneously targeting BCMA and GPRC5D to prevent BCMA escape–driven relapse in multiple myeloma. Blood Cancer Discovery. 2020;1(2):146–54.

Gardner R, Wu D, Cherian S, Fang M, Hanafi LA, Finney O, et al. Acquisition of a CD19-negative myeloid phenotype allows immune escape of MLL-rearranged B-ALL from CD19 CAR-T cell therapy. Blood. 2016;127(20):2406–10.

de Haart SJ, van de Donk NW, Minnema MC, Huang JH, Aarts-Riemens T, Bovenschen N, et al. Accessory cells of the microenvironment protect multiple myeloma from T-cell cytotoxicity through cell adhesion-mediated immune resistance. Clin Cancer Res. 2013;19(20):5591–601.

de Haart SJ, Holthof L, Noort WA, Minnema MC, Emmelot ME, Aarts-Riemens T, et al. Sepantronium bromide (YM155) improves daratumumab-mediated cellular lysis of multiple myeloma cells by abrogation of bone marrow stromal cell-induced resistance. Haematologica. 2016;101(8):e339–42.

Hanabuchi S, Koyanagi M, Kawasaki A, Shinohara N, Matsuzawa A, Nishimura Y, et al. Fas and its ligand in a general mechanism of T-cell-mediated cytotoxicity. Proc Natl Acad Sci. 1994;91(11):4930–4.

Holthof L, van der Schans J, Katsarau A, Poels R, Gelderloos A, van Hal SE, et al. Bone marrow mesenchymal stromal cells can render multiple myeloma cells resistant to cytotoxic machinery of CAR-T cells through inhibition of apoptosis. Clin Cancer Res. 2021a;27(13):3793–803.

Holthof L, van der Horst HJ, Gelderloos A, Poels R, Li F, Groen R, et al. Bone marrow mesenchymal stromal cell-mediated resistance in multiple myeloma against NK cells can be overcome by introduction of CD38-CAR or TRAIL-variant. Hema. 2021b;5(5):e561.

Jain MD, Zhao H, Wang X, Atkins R, Menges M, Reid K, et al. Tumor interferon signaling and suppressive myeloid cells associate with CAR-T cell failure in large B cell lymphoma. Blood. 2021;137(19):2621–33.

Jilani I, O'Brien S, Manshuri T, Thomas DA, Thomazy VA, Imam M, et al. Transient down-modulation of CD20 by rituximab in patients with chronic lymphocytic leukemia. Blood. 2003;102(10):3514–20.

Karlsson SCH, Lindqvist AC, Fransson M, Paul-Wetterberg G, Nilsson B, Essand M, et al. Combining CAR-T cells and the Bcl-2 family apoptosis inhibitor ABT-737 for treating B-cell malignancy. Cancer Gene Ther. 2013;20(7):386–93.

Leblay N, Maity R, Barakat E, McCulloch S, Duggan P, Jimenez-Zepeda V, et al. Cite-Seq profiling of T cells in multiple myeloma patients undergoing BCMA targeting CAR-T or bites immunotherapy. Blood. 2020;136(Suppl 1):11–2.

McMillin DW, Delmore J, Negri JM, Vanneman M, Koyama S, Schlossman RL, et al. Compartment-specific bioluminescence imaging platform for the high-throughput evaluation of antitumor immune function. Blood. 2012;119(15):e131–8.

Moon EK, Wang LC, Dolfi DV, Wilson CB, Ranganathan R, Sun J, et al. Multifactorial T-cell hypofunction that is reversible can limit the efficacy of chimeric antigen receptor-transduced human T cells in solid tumors. Clin Cancer Res. 2014;20(16):4262–73.

Munshi NC, Anderson LD Jr, Shah N, Madduri D, Berdeja J, Lonial S, et al. Idecabtagene Vicleucel in relapsed and refractory multiple myeloma. N Engl J Med. 2021;384(8):705–16.

Neelapu SS, Locke FL, Bartlett NL, Lekakis LJ, Miklos DB, Jacobson CA, et al. Axicabtagene ciloleucel CAR-T cell therapy in refractory large B-cell lymphoma. N Engl J Med. 2017;377(26):2531–44.

Neelapu SS, Rossi JM, Jacobson CA, Locke FL, Miklos DB, Reagan PM, et al. CD19-loss with preservation of other B cell lineage features in patients with large B cell lymphoma who relapsed post-axi-cel. Blood. 2019;134(Suppl 1):203.

Orlando EJ, Han X, Tribouley C, Wood PA, Leary RJ, Riester M, et al. Genetic mechanisms of target antigen loss in CAR19 therapy of acute lymphoblastic leukemia. Nat Med. 2018;24(10):1504–6.

Paul MR, Wong V, Aristizabal P, Kuo DJ. Treatment of recurrent refractory pediatric pre-B acute lymphoblastic leukemia using Inotuzumab Ozogamicin monotherapy resulting in CD22 antigen expression loss as a mechanism of therapy resistance. J Pediatr Hematol Oncol. 2019;41(8):e546–e9.

Plesner T, van de Donk N, Richardson PG. Controversy in the use of CD38 antibody for treatment of myeloma: is high CD38 expression good or bad? Cell. 2020;9(2):378.

Rasche L, Hudecek M, Einsele H. What is the future of immunotherapy in multiple myeloma? Blood. 2020;136(22):2491–7.

Samur MK, Fulciniti M Aktas-Samur A, Hamid Bazarbachi A, Tai Y, Campbell TB, Petrocca F, Hege K, Kaiser S, Anderson K, Munshi NC (2020) Biallelic loss of BCMA triggers resistance to anti-BCMA CAR-T cell therapy in multiple myeloma (abstract #721). 62nd ASH annual meeting and exposition

van der Schans JJ, van de Donk N, Mutis T. Dual targeting to overcome current challenges in multiple myeloma CAR-T cell treatment. Front Oncol. 2020;10:1362.

Singh N, Lee YG, Shestova O, Ravikumar P, Hayer KE. Impaired death receptor signaling in leukemia causes antigen-independent resistance by inducing CAR-T cell dysfunction. 2020;10(4):552–67.

Sotillo E, Barrett DM, Black KL, Bagashev A, Oldridge D, Wu G, et al. Convergence of acquired mutations and alternative splicing of CD19 enables resistance to CART-19 immunotherapy. Cancer Discov. 2015;5(12):1282–95.

Srivastava S, Furlan SN, Jaeger-Ruckstuhl CA, Sarvothama M, Berger C, Smythe KS, et al. Immunogenic chemotherapy enhances recruitment of CAR-T cells to lung tumors and improves antitumor efficacy when combined with checkpoint blockade. Cancer Cell. 2021;39(2):193–208.e10.

Sutton VR, Davis JE, Cancilla M, Johnstone RW, Ruefli AA, Sedelies K, et al. Initiation of apoptosis by granzyme B requires direct cleavage of bid, but not direct granzyme B-mediated caspase activation. J Exp Med. 2000;192(10):1403–14.

Textor A, Listopad JJ, Wuhrmann LL, Perez C, Kruschinski A, Chmielewski M, et al. Efficacy of CAR-T cell therapy in large tumors relies upon stromal targeting by IFNgamma. Cancer Res. 2014;74(23):6796–805.

Yang M, Wang L, Ni M, Schubert M-L, Neuber B, Hückelhoven-Krauss A, et al. The effect of apoptosis inhibitor blockade agents on the third generation CD19 CAR-T cells. Blood. 2019;134(Suppl 1):5620.

CART Initiatives in Europe

5

Alvaro Urbano-Ispizua and Michael Hudecek

The efficacy of chimeric antigen receptor T cells (CARTs) in B cell neoplasms, ALL, large B cell lymphoma, and now multiple myeloma has been one of the great achievements in the fight against cancer in recent decades (Porter et al. 2011). However, there is still a need to increase the proportion of responses (especially in NHL) (Locke et al. 2019) and to decrease the proportion of relapse (especially in ALL) (Grupp et al. 2013). More importantly, currently, commercial CAR-T products are not available for T cell neoplasms, myeloid malignant haemopathies, or solid tumours. As a reflection of the necessary efforts to expand the efficacy of CARTs, more than 500 clinical trials are currently underway worldwide, mostly led by American or Chinese groups. Unfortunately, European institutions are underrepresented in these initiatives. It is our duty to push and harmonize European academic clinical trials. We identified 35 early clinical trials promoted by European groups in Eudract and ClinTrialsGov (20 February 2021) (Table 5.1). Among them, 20 are initiatives from academic institutions, and 15 are initiatives from European companies allied with European academic institutions. In this summary, CART clinical trials promoted by European academic centres or by small to medium European companies are listed. The aim is to inform European groups treating haemato-oncology diseases of the current situation in this field, facilitating the inclusion of patients in these clinical trials. We aim to support the groups promoting these studies to increase collaboration.

A. Urbano-Ispizua
Institute of Hematology and Oncology. Hospital Clinic of Barcelona. University of Barcelona, Barcelona, Spain
e-mail: aurbano@clinic.cat

M. Hudecek (✉)
Department of Internal Medicine II, University Hospital of Würzburg, Würzburg, Germany
e-mail: Hudecek_M@ukw.de

© The Author(s) 2022
N. Kröger et al. (eds.), *The EBMT/EHA CAR-T Cell Handbook*,
https://doi.org/10.1007/978-3-030-94353-0_5

Table 5.1 Ongoing CART clinical trials in Europe

Title	Clinical Trial Gov Identifier	EudraCT Number	Institution	Target	Age Population	Disease
EUROPEAN CLINICAL TRIALS PROMOTED BY ACADEMIC CENTER						
Evaluation of CAR19 T-cells as an Optimal Bridge to Allogeneic Transplantation (COBALT)	NCT02431988	2015-000348-40	University College London	CD19	all ages	NHL DLBC
CAR19 Donor Lymphocytes for Relapsed CD19+ Malignancies Following Allogeneic Transplantation (CARD)	NCT02893189		University College London	CD19	Adult	CD19+ diseases
CARPALL: Immunotherapy With CD19 CAR T-cells for CD19+ Haematological Malignancies	NCT02443831		University College London	CD19	Pediatric	ALL
Immunotherapy with CD19ζ CAR gene-modified EBV-specific CTLs after stem cell transplant in children with high-risk ALL	NCT01195480	2007-007612-29	University College London	CD19	Pediatric	ALL
Phase 1, open label study of CRISPR-CAR genome edited T cells (TT52CAR19) in R/R B Cell ALL		2019-003462-40	Great Ormond Street Hospital	CD19	Pediatric	ALL
A Cancer Research UK Phase I Trial of Anti-GD2 CAR Transduced T-cells (1RG-CART) in Patients With R/R Neuroblastoma	NCT02761915		Great Ormond Street Hospital/CaResearchUK	GD2	all ages	Neuroblastoma
Phase I Trial: T4 Immunotherapy of Head and Neck Cancer	NCT01818323		King's College London	ErbB receptor	Adult	Head and Neck Cancer
Phase I Study for the Adoptive Transfer of Re-directed FAP-specific T Cells in the Pleural Effusion of Patients With Malignant Pleural Mesothelioma.	NCT01722149		University of Zurich	FAP	Adult	Mesothelioma
Targeting Leukemic Stem Cell Expressing the IL-1RAP Protein in CML	NCT02842320		Centre Hospitalier Universitaire de Besancon	IL-1RAP	Adult	CML
Phase I/II Study of Anti-GD2 CAR-Expressing T Cells in Pediatric Patients Affected by High Risk and/or R/R Neuroblastoma or Other GD2-positive Solid Tumors	NCT03373097	2017-002475-26	Bambino Gesù Hospital and Research Institute	GD2	Pediatric	Neuroblastoma
Phase I/II Study of Anti-CD19 Chimeric Antigen Receptor-Expressing T Cells in Pediatric Patients Affected by R/R CD19+ ALL and NHL	NCT03373071	2017-002088-16	Bambino Gesù Hospital and Research Institute	CD19	Pediatric	CD19+ diseases
Phase 1-2a Trial to Determine the Feasibility and Safety of a Single Dose of Transposon-manipulated AlloCARCIK-CD19 Cells in R/R B-cell ALL, After HSCT	NCT03389035	2017-000900-38	Fondazione Matilde Tettamanti Menotti De Marchi Onlus	CD19	all ages	ALL
Pilot Study on the Infusion of Differentiated Autologous T-cells with Anti-CD19 Specificity CAR (ARI0001)in Patients With R/R CD19+ Leukemia or Lymphoma	NCT03144583	2016-002972-29	Hospital Clínic Barcelona	CD19	all ages	CD19+ diseases

	NCT	EudraCT	Institution/Company	Target	Age	Indication
Clinical Trial Using Humanized CART Directed Against BCMA (ARIO002h) in Patients With Relapsed/Refractory Multiple Myeloma to Proteasome Inhibitors, Immunomodulators and Anti-CD38 Antibody	NCT04309981	2019-001472-11	Hospital Clinic Barcelona	BCMA	Adult	MM
Phase 2 Study of the Infusion of ARI-0001 Cells in Patients With CD19 + Acute Lymphoid Leukemia Resistant or Refractory to Therapy (CART19-BE-02)	NCT04778579		Hospital Clinic Barcelona	CD19	Adult	ALL
Immunotherapy with differentiated Tlymphocytes genetically modified to express a chimeric receptor with anti-CD30 specificity in patients with classic Hodgkin's lymphoma and NHL-T CD30+		2019-001263-70	IIBSP-Sant Pau Hospital	CD30	Adult	Hodgkin lymphoma and T-NHL CD30+
CD19-targeting 3rd generation CAR T cells for refractory B cell malignancy - a phase I/IIa trial.	NCT03068416	2013-001393-19	Uppsala University	CD19	all ages	CD19+ diseases
Treatment of patients with R/R CD19+ lymphoid disease with T lymphocytes transduced by RV-SFG.CD19.CD28.4-1BBzeta retroviral vector - A unicenter Phase I /II clinical trial	NCT03676504	2016-004808-60	University Hospital Heidelberg	CD19	all ages	CD19+ diseases
CD19-targeting 3rd generation CAR T cells for refractory B cell malignancy - a phase I/IIa trial. A phase II trial.		2016-004043-36	Uppsala University	CD19	all ages	CD19+ diseases
A phase I/IIa clinical trial to assess feasibility, safety and antitumor activity of autologous SLAMF7 CAR-T cells in MM	NCT04499339	2019-001264-30	Universitätsklinikum Würzburg	SLAMF7	Adult	MM
EUROPEAN CLINICAL TRIALS PROMOTED BY EUROPEAN COMPANIES						
A Phase I-IIa trial to assess the safety and antitumor activity of autologous CD44v6 CAR T-cells in AML and MM expressing CD44v6.	NCT04097301	2018-000813-19	MolMed S.p.A.	CD44v6	all ages	MM
A Single-Arm, Open-Label, Multi-Centre, Phase I/II Study Evaluating the Safety and Clinical Activity Of AUTO3, a CAR T Cell Treatment Targeting CD19 And CD22 in Paediatric And Young Adult Patients With R/R -ALL	NCT03289455	2016-004680-39	Autolus Limited	CD19/CD22	Pediatric	ALL
A Single Arm, Open-label, Multi-centre, Phase I/II Study Evaluating the Safety and Clinical Activity of AUTO3, a CAR T Cell Treatment Targeting CD19 and CD22 With Anti PD1 Antibody in Patients With R/R DLBCL	NCT03287817	2016-004682-11	Autolus Limited	CD19/CD22	Adult	HNL DLBC
A Single Arm, Open-Label, Multi-centre, Phase I/II Study Evaluating the Safety And Clinical Activity of AUTO4, a CAR T CELL Treatment Targeting TRBC1, in patients With R/R TRBC1 Positive Selected T cell NHL	NCT03590574	2017-001965-26	Autolus Limited	TRBC1	Adult	T-NHL
A Single Arm, Open-Label, Multi-Centre, Phase I/II Study Evaluating the Safety and Clinical Activity of AUTO3, a CAR T Cell Treatment Targeting CD19 and CD22 with Anti PD-1 Antibody in Patients with R/R DLBCL		2016-004682-11	Autolus Limited	CD19/CD22	Adult	HNL DLBC
A Single Arm, Open-Label, Multi-Centre, Phase I/II Study Evaluating the Safety and Clinical Activity of AUTO2, a CAR T Cell Treatment Targeting BCMA and TACI, in Patients with R/R MM	NCT03287804	2016-003893-42	Autolus Limited	CD19	Adult	MM
An Open-Label, Multi-Centre, Phase Ib/II Study Evaluating The Safety and Efficacy Of AUTO1, A CAR T Cell Treatment Targeting CD19, In Adult Patients With R/ R B-ALL.	NCT04404660	2019-001937-16	Autolus Limited	CD19	Adult	ALL

(continued)

Table 5.1 (continued)

Title	Clinical Trial Gov Identifier	EudraCT Number	Institution	Target	Age Population	Disease
An Open-label, Phase I Study to Assess the Safety of Multiple Doses of CYAD-101, Administered After Standard FOLFOX or FOLFIRI Chemotherapy in Patients With Unresectable Metastatic Colorectal Cancer	NCT03692429		Celyad	NKG2D	Adult	Colorectal Cancer
A phase 1, open label, non-comparative, study to evaluate the safety and the ability of UCART19 to induce molecular remission in paediatric patients with relapsed /refractory B-cell acute lymphoblastic leukaemia		2015-004293-15	Servier	CD19	Pediatric	ALL
A phase I, Open Label, Dose-escalation Study Followed by a Safety Expansion Part to Evaluate the Safety, Expansion and Persistence of a Single Dose of UCART19 in Patients With R/R B-ALL	NCT02746952	2016-000296-24	Servier	CD19	Adult	ALL
Multicenter Phase I Trial of MB-CART20.1 for the Treatment of Patients With Metastatic Melanoma	NCT03893019		Miltenyi Biotec GmbH	CD20	Adult	Melanoma
A Phase I/II Safety, Dose Finding and Feasibility Trial of MB-CART20.1 in Patients With Relapsed or Resistant CD20 Positive B-NHL	NCT03664635		Miltenyi Biotec GmbH	CD19	Adult	NHL DLBC
A Phase I/II Safety, Dose Finding and Feasibility Trial of MB-CART19.1 in Patients With Relapsed or Refractory CD19 Positive B Cell Malignancies	NCT03853616	2017-002848-32	Miltenyi Biotec GmbH	CD19	all ages	CD19+ diseases
Phase I, open label dose-escalation study to evaluate the safety, expansion, persistence and clinical activity of multiple infusions of UCART123 in patients with adverse genetic risk AML		2018-001018-14	CELLECTIS SA Fr	CD123	Adult	AML
Assessing Feasibility of Expansion and Characterization of Gamma Delta T Cells of Patients With AML as Starting Product for Generation of CD33-CD28 Gamma Delta T Cells	NCT03885076		Royal Marsden NHS/TC Biopharm	CD33	Adult	AML
Phase I/IIa, First-in-human (FIH), Open-label, Dose Escalation Trial With Expansion Cohorts to Evaluate Safety and Preliminary Efficacy of CLDN6 CAR-T +/- CLDN6 RNA-LPX in Patients With CLDN6-positive Relapsed or Refractory Advanced Solid Tumors	NCT04503278	2019-004323-20	BioNTech Cell & Gene Therapies GmbH	CLDN6	Adult	Solid tumor

Abbreviations: R/R, relapsed/refractory; ALL, aute lymphoblastic leukemia; AML, acute myeloblastic leukemia; MM, multiple myeloma; NHL, non hodgkin lymphoma; DLBCL, diffuse large B cell lymphoma; CML, chronic myeloid leukemia; HSCT, hemopoetic stem cell transplantation

Twelve European institutions are responsible for the 20 academic clinical trials (University College London, $n = 4$; Hospital Clinic of Barcelona, $n = 3$; Great Ormond Street Hospital, $n = 2$; Bambino Gesù, $n = 2$; University of Uppsala, $n = 2$; King's College, $n = 1$; Matilde Tettamanti, $n = 1$; Hospital Sant Pau, $n = 1$; University of Heidelberg, $n = 1$; and University of Wurzburg, $n = 1$). The most frequent target is CD19 ($n = 12$; for ALL, $n = 5$; NHL, $n = 1$; all B-lymphoid neoplasms, $n = 6$). Other targets are BCMA ($n = 1$; MM), CD30 ($n = 1$; HL and T-NHL), SLAMF7 ($n = 1$; MM), GD2 ($n = 2$, neuroblastoma), ErbBR ($n = 1$, neck and head tumours), Fap ($n = 1$, mesothelioma), and IL-1 RAP ($n = 1$, CML). Of the 20 clinical trials, 8 only included adults, 5 only included children, and 7 included all ages.

There were 16 additional clinical trials promoted by seven European pharma companies (Autolous, $n = 6$; Miltenyi, $n = 3$; Servier, $n = 2$; MolMed, $n = 1$; Celyad, $n = 1$; Cellectis, $n = 1$; TcBiopharm, $n = 1$, BioNTech, $n = 1$). Again, the most frequent target is CD19 ($n = 4$; for ALL, $n = 2$; NHL, $n = 1$; all B-lymphoid neoplasms, $n = 1$). Other targets are dual CD19/CD20 or CD19/CD22 ($n = 3$; ALL, $n = 1$; NHL, $n = 2$), CD20 ($n = 2$; melanoma, lymphoma), BCMA ($n = 1$; MM), CD123 ($n = 1$; AML), CD33 ($n = 1$, AML), NKG2D ($n = 1$, colon cancer), CD44v6 ($n = 1$, MM), TRCDB1 ($n = 1$, T-NHL), and CLDN6 ($n = 1$; colon cancer).

Hopefully, this list will grow as more clinical trials are set up. We intend to compile an ad hoc workshop to provide more comprehensive data, such as the characteristics of the genetic construct (type of costimulatory molecule, 2nd- or third-generation CAR), the vector (viral or nonviral), and the method of expansion (automated or manual) and the plans of these groups to go beyond a particular clinical trial (hospital exemption, EMA). We believe this information will be useful to increase efforts and fuel this field in Europe.

Two initiatives have recently been launched to foster collaboration and increase CART activity in Europe: GoCART and T2 EVOLVE Consortium.

GoCART is a strategic partnership between EBMT and EHA that includes a multistakeholder coalition of patient representatives, health care professionals, pharmaceutical companies, regulators, health technology assessment (HTA) bodies, reimbursement agencies, and medical organizations. Some of its most important aims include the following:

- Collaborate and share data and knowledge.
- Promote harmonization of data collection, education, standards of care, regulatory approval, centre qualification, and reimbursement processes.
- Set up a pre- and postmarketing registry that supports regulatory and shared research purposes.
- Develop a cellular therapy education and information program for patients and health care professionals.

T2EVOLVE is an alliance of academic and industry leaders in cancer immunotherapy under the European Union's Innovative Medicines Initiative (Supported from the European Union's Horizon 2020 Research and Innovation Programme). The key objective of T2EVOLVE is to accelerate development and increase the awareness and access of cancer patients to immunotherapy with immune cells that harbour a genetically engineered TCR or CAR. Simultaneously, T2EVOLVE aims to provide guidance on sustainable integration of these treatments into the EU health care system. The T2EVOLVE consortium aims to achieve its goal by working on and improving the state of the art in the following key aspects:

- Selection of optimal lymphodepletion regimens.
- Optimization of preclinical models for the best safety and efficacy prediction.
- To involve and guide patients throughout their clinical journey.
- Definition of gold standard analytical methods pre- and post-engineered T cell infusion.
- Production of GMP guidance and establishment of standard product profiles.
- To produce excellent cancer therapies accessible to all European patients.

Key Points
1. Two initiatives have been launched to foster collaboration and increase CART activity in Europe: GoCART and T2 EVOLVE Consortium.
2. A large number of CAR-T cell clinical trials are underway.
3. Most clinical trials are occurring in the USA and China, and although Europe has lagged behind, there is evidence of increasing activity.
4. Initiatives to enhance clinical trial activity and cooperation across Europe are needed, and various initiatives are planned to facilitate this.

References

Grupp SA, Kalos M, Barrett D, et al. Chimeric antigen receptor–modified T cells for acute lymphoid leukemia. N Engl J Med. 2013;368:1509–18.
Locke FL, Ghobadi A, Jacobson CA, et al. Long-term safety and activity of axicabtagene ciloleucel in refractory large B-cell lymphoma (ZUMA-1): a single-arm, multicentre, phase 1–2 trial. Lancet Oncol. 2019;20:31–42. https://doi.org/10.1016/S1470-2045(18)30864-7.
Porter DL, Levine BL, Kalos M, et al. Chimeric antigen receptor–modified T cells in chronic lymphoid leukemia. N Engl J Med. 2011;365:725–33.

Part II

Manufacturing CAR-T Cells: The Supply Chain

Providing the Starting Material to the Manufacturer of an Approved and Commercially Available Autologous CAR-T Cell Treatment

6

Halvard Bonig, Christian Chabannon (iD), and Miquel Lozano

Introduction

CAR-T cell manufacturing starts from a collection of mononuclear cells (MNCs, although specifically only T lymphocytes will be used for the preparation) from the patient using apheresis. Although several initiatives are working on the development of allogeneic CAR-T cells, currently only CAR-T therapies of autologous origin are approved in the European Union. The present chapter only discusses already or soon-to-be marketed autologous CAR-T cells and excludes investigational CAR-T cells or rare CAR-T cells approved in the context of hospital exemption, such as the ARI-001 product (Ortiz-Maldonado et al. 2021); on this topic, please refer to Chap. 3.

Institutions aspiring to be CAR-T centres must generate sufficient apheresis capacity to ensure immediate access to apheresis slots; apheresis capacity must grow in synchrony with the CAR-T program (Tables 6.1, 6.2, 6.3, 6.4, and 6.5).

H. Bonig
Translational Development of Cellular Therapeutics, Institute for Transfusion Medicine and Immunohematology, Goethe University, Frankfurt, Germany

Medicine/Hematology, University of Washington, Seattle, WA, USA

Transfusion Medicine, University of Ljubljana, Ljubljana, Slovenia
e-mail: H.Boenig@blutspende.de

C. Chabannon (✉)
Institut Paoli-Calmettes, Centre de Lutte Contre le Cancer, Centre d'Investigations Cliniques en Biothérapie, Université d'Aix-Marseille, Inserm CBT-1409, Marseille, France
e-mail: CHABANNONC@ipc.unicancer.fr

M. Lozano
Department of Hemotherapy and Hemostasis, Institute of Hematology and Oncology, Clinic University Hospital, University of Barcelona, IDIBAPS, Barcelona, Catalonia, Spain
e-mail: MLOZANO@clinic.cat

31

N. Kröger et al. (eds.), *The EBMT/EHA CAR-T Cell Handbook*,
https://doi.org/10.1007/978-3-030-94353-0_6

Table 6.1 Before apheresis collection

Apheresis units might require a visit during the screening of patients for CAR-T therapies

In the visit the following aspects should be evaluated (Yakoub-Agha et al. 2020):
- Discontinue drugs that affect the number and functionality of circulating T lymphocytes (e.g., steroids, immune-suppressors, and chemotherapy) as long as possible before apheresis. Minimal stopping rules are defined in institutional guidelines and manufacturing authorization holder (MAH) instructions. Steroids are usually stopped at least 3–7 days before apheresis.
- Evaluate for systemic infection, particularly in patients with an intravenous central line. Bacteremia is a relative contraindication for MNC apheresis due to the risk of contamination of the product. Note, however, that a contaminated blood product—although definitely not ideal—is not always rejected by the manufacturer because the manufacturing process may plan for the addition of antibiotics.
- Assess venous access, ideally including an ultrasound evaluation if upper arm peripheral veins are not adequate by palpation (Gopalasingam et al. 2017) before deciding that a central line catheter must be placed. Blood can be collected from most adult patients via peripheral access sites. Central catheters are most often needed in low-weight children. Indwelling catheters are suitable (Jarisch et al. 2020).
- Evaluate whether any form of sedation is necessary (mostly for the paediatric population) through a joint evaluation between the paediatricians and apheresis medical director or practitioner.
- Review complete blood count (CBC) and differential (absolute lymphocyte count) results to calculate target process volume.
- Check the MCV to rule out the presence of beta thalassemia minor. Microcytosis leads to abnormal sedimentation behaviour, necessitating modification of apheresis settings (Constantinou et al. 2017).
- Note height and weight and calculate total blood volume. In particular, in low-weight children, consider the need for priming of the apheresis tubing set with irradiated red blood cell concentrate (which needs to be pre-ordered so as not to delay initiation of apheresis).
- If the patient is transfused with cellular components in the days prior to apheresis collection, they must be gamma irradiated.
- Note concurrent medications, especially anti-hypertensives. Angiotensin-converting enzyme inhibitors and beta-blockers increase the risk of hypotension reactions during apheresis.
- Evaluate electrolyte levels: potassium, (ionized) calcium, and magnesium levels drop during apheresis and thus can become critically low if already abnormal before apheresis (Stenzinger and Bonig 2018).
- Negative infectious markers of HIV, HBV, and HCV (in some countries also HTLV-1 and syphilis) must be available within 30 days of collection, in compliance with applicable laws and regulations for autologous cell products. MAH will require that results be available upon shipment of the starting material to the manufacturing site.

Table 6.2 Designing apheresis collection

– Select the apheresis platform suitable for the collection. Depending on the platform selected, the characteristics of the product collected might vary significantly. For instance, if an Amicus separator (Fresenius-Kabi, Bad Homburg, Germany) is used, the platelet content is very low in comparison to Spectra Optia (Terumo BCT, Lakewood, CO, USA) (Cid et al. 2019), see Table 6.3.
– Check if the total blood volume of the patient requires priming of the apheresis separator.
– Check lymphocyte count to define the blood volume to be processed, see Table 6.4 for apheresis targets of different manufacturers.
– Consider prophylactic administration of calcium and magnesium during the collection depending on the volume to be processed (Sörensen et al. 2013).
– Evaluate the haemoglobin and platelet count, consider transfusion prior to or after apheresis depending on circumstances. A haemoglobin level of 7 g/dL, better yet 8 g/dL, prior to apheresis facilitates establishment of interphase during apheresis. Spectra Optia will reduce platelet count by approximately 11% per total blood volume processed.
– Evaluate the potassium level and consider supplementation.

Table 6.3 Characteristics of the apheresis platforms typically used for collection

	Amicus	Spectra optia	
Manufacturer	Fresenius-Kabi (Bad Homburg, Germany)	TerumoBCT, Lakewood, Co, USA	
Software kit		Continuous MNC (CMNC)	MNC
Flow type	Discontinuous	Continuous	Dual-stage separation
Flow rate	10–80 (85) mL/min[a]	10–142 mL/min	10–125 mL/min
Operation	Automatic	Semi-automatic	Semi-automatic
Mononuclear cell collection	Elutriation	Aspiration	Aspiration followed by elutriation
Platelets	Returned to the donor	Collected	Partially returned to donor

[a]Depending on the leukocyte count

Table 6.4 Collection requirements of different manufacturers of CAR-T therapies

Product	Axicabtagene ciloleucel	Brexucabtagene autoleucel	Tisagenlecleucel	Lisocabtagene maraleucel	Idecabtagene vicleucel	Ciltacabtagene autoleucel
Registered name	Yescarta®	Tecartus®	Kymriah®	Breyanzi®	Abecma®	
Manufacturer	Gilead	Gilead	Novartis	Juno-Celgene-BMS	BlueBird Bio-Celgene-BMS	Legend Therapeutics-Janssen
Antigen recognized	CD19	CD19	CD19	CD19	BCMA	BCMA
Target cell dose during apheresis[a]	$5–10 \times 10^9$ MNCs		$1–4 \times 10^9$ CD3+ cells $\geq 2 \times 10^9$ TNCs $\geq 3\%$ CD3+ of TNCs (rounding rules apply)			
Target volume to be processed[a]	12–15 L		6–10 L			

[a]Manufacturer's recommendation

MNCs mononuclear cells, *TNCs* total nucleated cells

Table 6.5 Interim storage, cryopreservation, and logistics

• Interim storage at 4–8 °C

• Tisagenlecleucel: Adjust concentration to 10^8/mL (0.5–2×10^8); freeze as soon as feasible but no later than 24 h after collection, with DMSO as a cryoprotectant in a controlled-rate freezer; store in LN2 (institutional SOP to be validated by the manufacturer prior to start of operations).

• All other CAR-T cells: Ship as soon as possible at 4–8 °C, following the manufacturers' instructions and requirements.

• MAH to arrange pick-up, with temperature-controlled shipping containers of the appropriate temperature.

• Scheduling, documentation of pick-up, hand-over, and tracking supported by MAH-supplied specific web tools.

Key Points

• Prepare for apheresis by assessing the clinical and biological condition of the patient.

• Discontinue treatments that can lower immune effector cell numbers and functions.

• Tailor apheresis parameters to the patient condition.

• Tailor apheresis parameters to suit the manufacturer's needs and requirements.

• Tightly coordinate with the Cell Processing Facility to ensure smooth shipment to the manufacturing site, in compliance with the manufacturer's needs and requirements.

References

Cid J, Carbasse G, Alba C, Perea D, Lozano M. Leukocytapheresis in nonmobilized donors for cellular therapy protocols: evaluation of factors affecting collection efficiency of cells. J Clin Apher. 2019;34:672–9.

Constantinou VC, Bouinta A, Karponi G, et al. Poor stem cell harvest may not always be related to poor mobilization: lessons gained from a mobilization study in patients with beta-thalassemia major. Transfusion. 2017;57:1031–9.

Gopalasingam N, Thomsen AE, Folkersen L, Juhl-Olsen P, Sloth E. A successful model to learn and implement ultrasound-guided venous catheterization in apheresis. J Clin Apher. 2017;32:437–43.

Jarisch A, Rettinger E, Sorensen J, et al. Unstimulated apheresis for chimeric antigen receptor manufacturing in pediatric/adolescent acute lymphoblastic leukemia patients. J Clin Apher. 2020;35(5):398–405. https://doi.org/10.1002/jca.21812.

Ortiz-Maldonado V, Rives S, Castella M, et al. CART19-BE-01: a multicenter trial of ARI-0001 cell therapy in patients with CD19(+) relapsed/refractory malignancies. Mol Ther. 2021;29:636–44.

Sörensen J, Jarisch A, Smorta C, et al. Pediatric apheresis with a novel apheresis device with electronic interface control. Transfusion. 2013;53:761–5.

Stenzinger M, Bonig H. Risks of leukapheresis and how to manage them—a non-systematic review. Transfus Apher Sci. 2018;57:628–34.

Yakoub-Agha I, Chabannon C, Bader P, et al. Management of adults and children undergoing CAR-T cell therapy: best practice recommendations of the EBMT and JACIE. Haematologica. 2020;105:297–316.

Receiving, Handling, Storage, Thawing, Distribution, and Administration of CAR-T Cells Shipped from the Manufacturing Facility

7

Catherine Rioufol and Christian Wichmann

Definition

In the manufacturing process for antigen receptor T cell (CAR-T cell) therapies, the patient's T cells acquire medicinal product status after enrichment, genetic modification, and expansion.

This pharmacologic effect results from insertion of a transgene coding for CAR, recognizing the tumour antigen, lysing the tumour cells, and activating the immune system see Chaps. 1, 2 and 3 in Section 1. Moreover, CAR-T cells massively expand upon interaction with antigen-positive cells within the blood system, thereby increasing the number of administered ATMP cells to high numbers (June et al. 2018). Due to this pharmacologic mechanism, CAR-T cells, despite their cellular nature, are gene therapy medicinal products. Whether from patients or healthy donors, CAR-T cells belong to the class of advanced therapy medicinal products (ATMPs), as defined in Regulation EC N°1394/2007 of the European Parliament and in Directive 2009/120/EC of the Council of November 13, 2007 on ATMPs, amending Directive 2001/83/EC and Regulation N° 726/2004.

As a consequence of this medicinal status, CAR-T cells fall under the responsibility of the hospital pharmacist. The manufacturer ships the released drugs to the pharmacy of the treatment centre; the hospital pharmacist is responsible of each step: reception, handling, storage, thawing, and dispensation (Pinturaud et al. 2018), regardless of whether the CAR-T cells are on the market or being used experimentally in a clinical trial. In hospitals with a Cell Processing Facility, the pharmacy

C. Rioufol (✉)
Hospices Civils de Lyon, UCBL1, EA 3738 CICLY, Lyon, France
e-mail: catherine.rioufol@chu-lyon.fr

C. Wichmann
Department of Transfusion Medicine, Cell Therapeutics and Hemostaseology, University Hospital, LMU Munich, Munich, Germany
e-mail: Christian.Wichmann@med.uni-muenchen.de

© The Author(s) 2022
N. Kröger et al. (eds.), *The EBMT/EHA CAR-T Cell Handbook*,
https://doi.org/10.1007/978-3-030-94353-0_7

may elect to subcontract certain technical operations to the Cell Processing Facility, as defined in an internal agreement. The overall handling and working process must be compliant with legal requirements enforced by local and national health authorities, and with the technical requirements of the drug-producing company (checked through audits and training courses).

Workflow	Description of the process
Handling	– Handling of CAR-T cells according to ATMP requirements, ensuring product safety and health care worker protection. Personal protective equipment (PPE) to protect the handling team involved throughout the various stages of the 'CAR-T pathway' – 'CAR-T hospital pathway' is supervised by the pharmacist; the steps are defined by the pharmaceutical team in coordination with the medical and nursing teams of the Haematology Department to meet objectives and ease the patient's care pathway – Need of a reliable adapted quality assurance system with initial and continuous training programs for all those involved, and periodic assessment, in addition to the centre qualification by the pharmaceutical laboratories – At many centres, CAR-T cell products are managed by specialized oncology pharmaceutical teams involved in cancer patient monitoring and treatment, and in close contact with the oncology department – Staff training and on-site inspection conducted by the manufacturer – Process control through web-based communication tools, with access provided by the manufacturer
Reception and conformity check	Critical steps: – Treatment confirmation in the context of a multidisciplinary meeting that examines that the indication is consistent with the marketing approval/SmPC and that the patient condition is compatible with the expected safety profile of the CAR-T cells – The hospital pharmacist's order is placed with the manufacturer – Planification of the collection of the starting material through leukapheresis at the cell collection facility (which may be operated by the treating hospital or subcontracted to another hospital or a blood bank) – Shipment of the starting material from the cell processing facility, which works in close collaboration with the cell collection facility (the cell processing facility may be operated by the treating hospital or subcontracted to another hospital or a blood bank) – Turnaround time of 4–6 weeks between ordering and receiving to allow for manufacturing and transportation (based on the experience of the first active European centres) – Tracking of the consecutive steps of on-demand medicinal product manufacturing on the manufacturer's website, allowing the date and time of reception to be known in advance to mobilize the necessary human resources for reception without interruption of the cold chain – Usual presentation of CAR-T cells: bag or syringe for infusion, delivered in a dry-shipper (vapour phase nitrogen) at approximately −160 °C

Workflow	Description of the process
	– Reception of the dry-shipper in ventilated premises
	– Conformity check at reception with reception documents (travel documents, certificates of analysis and release, temperature logs, labels): Cryo-shipper check: no visible damage and/or leaks
	Opening of the metal cassette to fully inspect the frozen cell product
	Checking the completeness and accuracy of information printed on the CAR-T cell label: patient identity and drug identity. Proper labelling is key to maintain the Chain of Identity/Chain of Custody throughout the manufacturing process, up to administration of the medicinal product to the intended recipient
	– Back-up bag: whether a back-up bag is available at the manufacturer's site should be systematically stated in the reception documents. In case of nonconformity detected at reception, this information is very useful for the pharmacist and haematologists in determining the treatment strategy: a back-up bag enables timely administration within 48 h via replacement of the defective CAR-T cells
	– All retrieved information is entered on the manufacturer's website
	– Transfer of the CAR-T cells to a cryogenic recipient
	– Management of out-of-range temperature or other abnormalities: storage of CAR-T cells in quarantine and contact of the manufacturer for instructions
	– Final check of Out of Specifications (OOS)
	– Double control involving two members of the pharmacy team or one member each from the pharmacy and cell processing facility for reception, conformity checking, and transfer to the cryogenic recipient
Storage	– Storage in vapour phase nitrogen tanks. In hospitals with a cell processing facility, storage is possible in a dedicated nitrogen tank. Respective responsibilities are then defined in an agreement approved by the health authority
	– The cryogenic premises preferably contain several nitrogen tanks for back-up in case of dysfunction. Having several distinct tanks also allows CAR-T cells with market authorization to be distinguished from those used in clinical trials or from other ATMPs. The tanks are fed by a central filling tank, and filling should be automated and levels monitored in real time, with a 24/7 alarm at the lower threshold. Temperature courses must be regularly monitored, saved, and controlled
	– Nitrogen storage time: approximately 6 months
	– Prevention of burns and hypoxia accidents in handling the CAR-T cells in and out of the nitrogen in the cryogenic recipients: ventilated premises, with secure access reserved to trained and retrained personnel, no access alone to the cryogenic area, and an oculus in the door so that any incident can be detected from the outside. Oxygen levels at the floor are recorded in real time and displayed with visual and sound alarms at the hospital security station. The nitrogen storage symbol is displayed. First-aid procedures are set out, with pictograms inside and outside the premises
	– Protection of the staff: use of PPE to prevent burning via nitrogen contact (gloves with sleeves up to the elbow, protective glasses, a lab coat, and boots). Follow institutional standard operating procedures for liquid nitrogen handling
	– Organization: stand-by duty rotation implemented for nights, weekends, and holidays to enable intervention in case of any malfunction outside of pharmacy opening times
	Regular maintenance ensures good functioning of premises and tanks

In the Storage row, the Workflow cell contains:

7   14.007

N

Nitrogen

Workflow	Description of the process
Thawing	– After medicinal product recovery from the storage tank, a double check (four-eyes principle) is again necessary to avoid any error in administration: this includes a careful check of patient identity: name, birth date, apheresis-ID, and batch number
	– Check of concordance between the product and the haematologist's prescription: patient identity, CAR-T denomination, administration date
	– Check of the expiration date (even though CAR-T cells are stable over a period of several months at temperatures below −160 °C)
	– Beginning of the thawing once the haematologist has given the green light
	– Thawing operations:
	Performed by the pharmaceutical team on the day of administration, with as short a time as possible; this requires coordinated planning with the Haematology Department
	Conducted on the pharmacy premises (or in the cell processing facility if subcontracted), after double-wrapping the bag of CAR-T cells in a protective plastic bag in a clean room, in a dedicated 37 ± 2 °C water bath until all ice crystals have melted in the bag. Depending on local organization, a dry thaw method may also be used
	Recommendation: double-wrap the bag in a watertight plastic bag for thawing, to protect the bag of CAR-T cells and observe and control any solution leakage due to accidental piercing of the original bag that may have been overlooked at reception
	After thawing, the CAR-T cells are stable at room temperature for approximately 30 to 90 min, depending on the manufacturer (please refer to the SmPC and the manufacturer's instructions)
	– Usually, no processing step (wash, spin down, etc.) is required or allowed
	– Commercial products should not be sampled
Preparation	– In case of CAR-T cells requiring processing before dispensation, injection preparation in a pressurized preparation room with vertical laminar airflow with no air recycling is necessary to prevent the risk of microbiological contamination of the product and to minimize risks to personnel and the environment
Transport to the Haematology departmen t	– The interval between thawing and administration is 30 to 90 min, depending on the manufacturer, requiring precise timing, including transport of the cells from the pharmacy to the department in a dedicated and clearly identified container at room temperature
	Warning: it is especially important to adhere to the manufacturer's recommended interval as it seems to be a question of the presence of dimethyl sulfoxide (DMSO), a cryopreservation agent that impairs cell quality and viability at room temperature, in the CAR-T cell medium (Li et al. 2019)
	– In most cases, due to the short lifespan of CAR-T cells after thawing and the risk of patient death in case of failure to administer, transport by the pharmacist or a member of the pharmacy staff is recommended
Dispensing in the Haematology Departmen t	– Dispensation under a ready-to-administer form from the pharmacy, preferably to the nurse who will be in charge of injection in the Haematology Department. Recording the dispensation time
	– Check by the pharmacist that the nurse has all the specific administration devices, notably including a non-leukodepleting in-line filter
	– All material that has been in contact with the CAR-T cell product (solid and liquid waste) should be handled and disposed of as potentially infectious waste and genetically modified organisms (GMOs) in accordance with local biosafety guidelines and local and national regulations

Administration

Five to seven days ahead of CAR-T cell injection, lymphodepleting chemotherapy is started (Maus and June 2016). It is recommended to await reception and conformity checking of the CAR-T ATMP to avoid unnecessarily reducing patient lymphocyte levels in cases where nonconformity prevents administration.

CAR-T cell administration is scheduled by the haematology department in coordination with the pharmacy team and the Cell Processing Facility to allow for completion of the circuit under optimal conditions without delay of administration. Patient information and consent for the entire CAR-T process, including CAR-T cell infusion, is provided in advance by haematologists.

The cells are delivered intravenously at a 10–20 mL/min infusion rate (gravity flow) without prewarming through a peripheral or central catheter. A non-leukodepleting in-line filter is used.

At some centres, the pharmacist is present at the bedside to respond to any request by the nurse, such as for an extra device. Even if not physically present, the pharmacist must remain quickly available upon request.

The hospital stay is approximately 2 weeks but longer in cases of major adverse events, such as cytokine release syndrome (CRS) or neurotoxicity, which may require transfer to the intensive care unit. Another important responsibility that lays with the hospital pharmacy is to ensure that two doses of tocilizumab (anti-IL-6R antibody) are immediately available for each treated patient as per SmPC.

Patients Treated with CAR-T Cells: New Missions for the Hospital Pharmacist

The steps along the CAR-T pathway highlight the role of the hospital pharmacist in this therapeutic innovation.

In the future, the increasing number and variety of ATMPs may require significant changes in pharmacy organization, notably in terms of premises and equipment (e.g., nitrogen tanks and vertical laminar airflow hoods) for proper and safe handling of the various types of ATMPs: somatic cell therapy medicinal products, gene therapy medicinal products (including CAR-T cells), and other categories of ATMPs, such as acellular gene therapy medicinal products, tissue engineering products, and combined medicinal products.

> **Key Points**
> - High medicinal standards of cell therapy products supervised by hospital pharmacists.
> - Cryopreservation: a strictly regulated working environment that ensures safety of the products and requires implementation of stringent measures to protect the physical safety of involved staff.

- High technical requirements, including 24/7 monitoring of the cell storage site.
- Patient pathway: plan lymphodepletion chemotherapy after reception of CAR-T cells.
- Statement in the reception document regarding whether a back-up bag is available.
- Overall, the process is conducted within different facilities and requires good communication skills and a multidisciplinary approach.

References

Commission Directive 2009/120/EC of 14 September 2009 amending Directive 2001/83/CE of the European Parliament and of the Council on the Community code relating to medicinal products for human use as regards Advanced Therapy Medicinal Products (text with EEA relevance).

June CH, O'Connor RS, Kawalekar OU, Ghassemi S, Milone MC. CAR-T cell immunotherapy for human cancer. Science. 2018;359(6382):1361–5. https://doi.org/10.1126/science.aar6711.

Li R, Johnson R, Yu G, McKenna DH, Hubel A. Preservation of cell-based immunotherapies for clinical trials. Cytotherapy. 2019;21(9):943–57. Epub 2019 Aug 12. PMID: 31416704; PMCID: PMC6746578. https://doi.org/10.1016/j.jcyt.2019.07.004.

Maus MV, June CH. Making better chimeric antigen receptors for adoptive T-cell therapy. Clin Cancer Res. 2016;22(8):1875–84. https://doi.org/10.1158/1078-0432.CCR-15-1433.

Pinturaud M, Vasseur M, Odou P. Role of the hospital pharmacist in the management of a category of advanced therapy medicinal product: chimeric antigen receptor T-cells. Bull Cancer. 2018;105:S205–13.

Regulation (EC) N° 1394/2007 of the European Parliament and of the Council of 13 November 2007 on Advanced Therapy Medicinal Products and amending Directive 2001/83/EC and Regulation (EC) n°726/2004 (text with EEA relevance), vol 324, 2007. http://data.europa.eu/eli/reg/2007/1394/oj/fra

Point-of-Care Production of CAR-T Cells

8

Julio Delgado, Claire Roddie, and Michael Schmitt

CAR-T cells for clinical application are classified as advanced therapy medicinal products (ATMPs), and their manufacture is subject to laws and regulations governed by the European Medicines Agency (EMA) and by federal and regional authorities. CAR-T cells must be manufactured to achieve good manufacturing practice (GMP) compliance and are defined as potent products manufactured safely according to standardized methods under closely controlled, reproducible, and auditable conditions. BioPharma supplies the vast majority of CAR-T products for patients, but some academic centres have developed point-of-care cGMP CAR-T manufacturing capability, striving to uphold the same stringency of product quality while improving patient access to CAR-T cells and streamlining the costs of therapy. Point-of-care CAR-T manufacturing can only be performed in facilities with the appropriate regulatory approvals in place.

J. Delgado
Department of Haematology, Hospital Clinic of Barcelona, Barcelona, Spain
e-mail: JDELGADO@clinic.cat

C. Roddie (✉)
University College London Cancer Institute, London, UK
e-mail: c.roddie@ucl.ac.uk

M. Schmitt
Medizinische Klinik (Krehl-Klinik), Zentrum für Innere Medizin, Klinik für Hämatologie, Onkologie und Rheumatologie, Innere Medizin V, Heidelberg, Germany
e-mail: michael.schmitt@med.uni-heidelberg.de

© The Author(s) 2022
N. Kröger et al. (eds.), *The EBMT/EHA CAR-T Cell Handbook*,
https://doi.org/10.1007/978-3-030-94353-0_8

GMP Vector Production

Retroviral and lentiviral vectors are the most common gene delivery methods used in CAR-T manufacture. Viral vectors are considered an intermediate reagent by regulatory agencies, but in manufacturing, adherence to cGMP conditions is recommended.

Vector manufacture is conducted in grade A laminar flow cabinets in grade B clean rooms, commonly using HEK293T packaging cell lines derived from a master cell bank (MCB), assuming the appropriate licencing agreements with Rockfeller University are in place. Quality control of the MCB is outlined in Table 8.1 (Perpiñá et al. 2020).

Nonviral techniques for gene transduction or gene-editing are under investigation in preclinical and early clinical trials (Prommersberger et al. 2021).

The vector manufacturing process takes 10 to 14 days and is outlined here. Packaging cells are expanded in flasks and transferred into cell culture chambers followed by plasmid transfection using polyethylenimine. Fixed quantities of plasmids encoding CAR, viral envelope, and gagpol are required. Following transfection, supernatants containing the secreted vector are harvested, clarified using 0.45-mm membranes, concentrated prior to diafiltration and cryopreservation in aliquots, and stored at -80 °C until use. Quality measures are outlined in Table 8.2 (Castellà et al. 2019).

Table 8.1 Quality control for the HEK293T master cell bank

Parameter	Method	Acceptance criteria
Appearance	Visual inspection	Presence of adherent cells with thin extensions
Sterility	Microbial growth	Sterile
Mycoplasma	PCR	Absent
Adventitious viruses	PCR	Absent
Karyotype	G-band staining	Informative
Cell viability (%) after thawing	Neubauer cell counting with trypan blue exclusion	>70%

Table 8.2 Quality control for GMP-grade virus production

Parameter	Method	Acceptance criteria
Appearance	Visual inspection	Yellowish liquid solution
Viral titre	Limiting dilution	$>3.75 \times 10^7$ TU/mL
Sterility	Microbial growth	Sterile
Mycoplasma	PCR	Absent
Identity	PCR	Positive
Replication-competent lentivirus	Real-time PCR	Absent

Manufacturing CAR-T Cells

CAR-T cell manufacturing is conducted over approximately 8–12 days in an approved cGMP clean room facility in a closed or functionally closed system to reduce the risk of product contamination (Roddie et al. 2019; Schubert et al. 2019; Castellá et al. 2020).

Starting material for CAR-T cells includes CD3+ T cells derived from nonmobilized leukapheresis (see Chap. 6). Mandated leukapheresis requirements of academic manufacturers for total nucleated cells (TNCs) and CD3+ T cells must be defined; as an illustration, the Uni. Heidelberg HD-CAR-1 protocol (EudraCT No. 2016-004808-60) requires 20×10^8 TNCs and 10×10^8 CD3+ T cells, similar to Novartis requirements for the manufacture of tisagenlecleucel. Leukapheresis material may be cryopreserved prior to manufacture, but in a bid to shorten the manufacturing process, there is a trend towards using fresh leukapheresis material. CAR-T manufacture is a stepwise process outlined in Table 8.3:

Upon completion of manufacturing, CAR-T products must comply with quality control/end-product specifications stipulated in the certificate of analysis. Parameters may vary, but CAR-T products are usually characterized for release according to

Table 8.3 CAR-T manufacturing methodology

	Potential methods	Timepoint
Step 1: T cell enrichment post-leukapheresis *(optional)*	Ficoll density gradient centrifugation; elutriation; immunomagnetic bead separation	Day 1
Step 2: T cell activation using synthetic antigen presenting technologies (CD3 +/− CD28) *(required)*	Soluble monoclonal antibodies; Para-magnetic anti-CD3/CD28 antibody coated beads; polymeric biodegradable CD3/28 incorporating nanomatrix (TransAct™)	Days 1, 2
Step 3: T cell stimulation *(required)*	IL-2, IL-7, and IL-15 in the culture medium (as per protocol) (Hoffmann et al. 2018; Gong et al. 2019)	From day 1 onwards
Step 4: Gene delivery/transduction with a retroviral or lentiviral CAR vector *(required)*	In some processes, retronectin or Vectofusin® is used to enhance transduction *(optional)*	Days 2, 3
Step 5: T cell expansion *(required)*	T-flasks, plates or culture bags; bioreactors, e.g., G-Rex™ flask (Wilson Wolf Manufacturing); Xuri WAVE™ Bioreactor (GE Life Systems); CliniMACS Prodigy™ (Miltenyi BioTec)	Days 3, 4 and onwards
Step 6: T cell harvest and cryopreservation *(required)*	The cryopreservation methodology often mirrors processes defined for haematopoietic cells. Methods include passive freezing (−80 °C freezer) and controlled-rate freezing	Day 8 onwards
Step 7: CAR-T cell quality assurance control and release testing	In-process and end of process controls are taken to ensure the product complies with release criteria specifications	Day 8 onwards

Table 8.4 Quality control of CAR-T cell biology and microbiology

Parameter	Method	Acceptance criteria
Appearance	Visual inspection	Cloudy liquid solution
CAR+ cells (%)[a]	Flow cytometry	>20%
CD3+ cells (%)	Flow cytometry	>70%
Cell viability (%)	Neubauer cell counting with trypan blue exclusion[b]	>70%
Sterility	Microbial growth E. Ph. 2.6.1	Sterile from bacteria/fungi
Mycoplasma	PCR[c]	Absent
Endotoxin	Chromogenic assay	<0.5 EU/mL
Optional/R&D		
CAR/CD45RA/CCR7 For detection of TE/ TEM/TEMRA/TCM/TN subpopulations	Flow cytometry	A high proportion of immature T cells is desirable for a long-lasting CAR-T cell effect in the patient
Cytotoxic potency	Cr-51 release assays in tumour CAR-T cell co-culture, assessed by flow cytometry	>40% killing at an effector/target ratio of 10:1 (or higher ratio) in a 4-h assay
Adventitious viruses	PCR	Absent
Number of transgene copies/cell	Real-time PCR (Kunz et al. 2019; Schubert et al. 2020)	<10 (range <7–15!) copies/cell[d]

[a]Automated cell counters, such as Luna™, are highly recommended
[b]Highly specific detection reagents (e.g., the Miltenyi Detection Reagent™) are strongly advised to distinguish CAR-T cells from the negative fraction
[c]European standards stipulate PCR methodology, in contrast to US regulations, which require serology
[d]Differs between countries and products

immunophenotypic, functional, and sterility assessments (Table 8.4). An out-of-specification (OOS) product cannot be released in the usual way, and its clinical use is at the discretion of the treating physician in concert with the regulatory authorities, informed through an OOS report.

> **Summary and Key Points**
> - Point-of-care/decentralized CAR-T cell manufacturing has the potential to enhance patient access to CAR-T products.
> - Limitations include the requirement for local cGMP facilities/trained staff and lack of standardization across multiple sites.
> - Potential solutions include implementation of standardized, semiautomated manufacturing platforms, such as the Miltenyi CliniMACS Prodigy™, and the use of standardized release assays reported in a common format across manufacturing sites to enable the manufacture of consistent, high-quality products between patients.

References

Castellà M, et al. Development of a novel anti-CD19 chimeric antigen receptor: a paradigm for an affordable CAR-T cell production at academic institutions. Mol Ther Methods Clin Dev. 2019;12:134–44.

Castellá M, et al. Point-of-care CAR-T cell production (ARI-0001) using a closed semi-automatic bioreactor: experience from an academic phase I clinical trial. Front Immunol. 2020;11:482.

Gong W, Hoffmann JM, Stock S, Wang L, Liu Y, Schubert ML, Neuber B, Hückelhoven-Krauss A, Gern U, Schmitt A, Müller-Tidow C, Shiku H, Schmitt M, Sellner L. Comparison of IL-2 vs IL-7/IL-15 for the generation of NY-ESO-1-specific T cells. Cancer Immunol Immunother. 2019;68(7):1195–209. Epub 2019 Jun 8. https://doi.org/10.1007/s00262-019-02354-4.

Hoffmann J-M, Schubert M-L, Wang L, Hückelhoven A, Sellner L, Stock S, Schmitt A, Kleist C, Gern A, Loskog A, Wuchter A, Hofmann S, Ho AD, Müller-Tidow C, Dreger P, Schmitt M. Differences in expansion potential of naive chimeric antigen receptor T cells from healthy donors and untreated chronic lymphocytic leukemia patients. Front Immunol. 2018;8:1956. https://doi.org/10.3389/fimmu.2017.01956.

Kunz A, Gern U, Schmitt A, Neuber N, Wang L, Hückelhoven-Krauss A, Michels B, Hofmann S, Müller-Tidow C, Dreger P, Schmitt M, Schubert M-L. Optimized assessment of qPCR-based vector copy numbers as a safety parameter for GMP-grade CAR-T cells and monitoring of frequency in patients. Mol Ther Methods Clin Dev. 2019;17:448–54.

Perpiñá U, et al. Cell banking of HEK293T cell line for clinical-grade lentiviral particles manufacturing. Transl Med Comm. 2020;5:22.

Prommersberger S, Reiser M, Beckmann J, Danhof S, Amberger M, Quade-Lyssy P, et al. CARAMBA: a first-in-human clinical trial with SLAMF7 CAR-T cells prepared by virus-free Sleeping Beauty gene transfer to treat multiple myeloma. Gene Ther. 2021;28(9):560–71. https://doi.org/10.1038/s41434-021-00254-w. Epub 2021 Apr 13. PMID: 33846552.

Roddie C, et al. Manufacturing chimeric antigen receptor T cells: issues and challenges. Cytotherapy. 2019;21(3):327–40. https://doi.org/10.1016/j.jcyt.2018.11.009.

Schubert M-L, Schmitt A, Sellner L, Neuber B, Kunz J, Wuchter P, Kunz A, Gern U, Michels B, Hofmann S, Hückelhoven-Krauss A, Kulozik A, Ho AD, Müller-Tidow C, Dreger P, Schmitt M. Treatment of patients with relapsed or refractory CD19+ lymphoid disease with T lymphocytes transduced by RV-SFG. CD19.CD28.4-1BBzeta retroviral vector: a unicentre phase I/II clinical trial protocol. BMJ Open. 2019;9:e026644. https://doi.org/10.1136/bmjopen-2018-026644.

Schubert ML, Kunz A, Schmitt A, Neuber B, Wang L, Hückelhoven-Krauss A, Langner S, Michels B, Wick A, Daniel V, Müller-Tidow C, Dreger P, Schmitt M. Assessment of CAR-T cell frequencies in Axicabtagene Ciloleucel and Tisagenlecleucel patients using duplex quantitative PCR. Cancers (Basel). 2020;12(10):2820.

Off-the-Shelf Allogeneic CAR-T Cells or Other Immune Effector Cells

9

Stephane Depil and Waseem Qasim

"Off-the-shelf" allogeneic CAR TCRαβ T cells and other immune effector cells, such as natural killer (NK) or gamma delta (gd) T cells, can be premanufactured from healthy donors and may offer alternatives to autologous strategies. However, major barriers, namely HLA disparity resulting in graft versus host disease (GvHD) and host-mediated rejection, must be addressed.

Strategies to Avoid Graft Versus Host Disease (GvHD)

Genome Edited αβTCR-Deleted T Cells

Strategies to reduce TCRαβ activity have included the use of truncated dominant-negative CD3ζ proteins (Gilham et al. 2018), protein expression blockers (PEBLs) (Kamiya et al. 2018), small hairpin RNA (Bunse et al. 2014), and genome editing. Platforms for the latter have included zinc-finger nucleases (ZFN) homing endonucleases/meganucleases, transcription activator-like effector nucleases (TALEN), megaTALs, clustered regularly interspaced short palindromic repeat (CRISP/cas9), and base editors (BEs) (Depil et al. 2020). Clinical trials of universal TCR-depleted CAR19 T cells produced using TALENs (Servier/Allogene) have been published (Qasim et al. 2017; Benjamin et al. 2020), and the first applications of meganuclease

S. Depil (✉)
Cancer Research Center of Lyon, Léon Bérard Cancer Center, University Claude Bernard Lyon 1, Lyon, France
e-mail: stephane.depil@lyon.unicancer.fr

W. Qasim
UCL Great Ormond Street Institute of Child Health, London, UK
e-mail: w.qasim@ucl.ac.uk

© The Author(s) 2022
N. Kröger et al. (eds.), *The EBMT/EHA CAR-T Cell Handbook*,
https://doi.org/10.1007/978-3-030-94353-0_9

(Precision Bio) and CRISPR engineering were recently reported (CRISPR Therapeutics). The manufacturing steps share common aspects of healthy donor T cell activation with anti-CD3/CD28 antibodies, editing by electroporation of nucleases and viral vector delivery of the CAR transgene. Depletion of residual TCRαβ T cells using a magnetic bead column ensures that the carriage of potentially alloreactive T cells is kept below the threshold that might lead to GvHD.

Virus-Specific T (VST) Cells

Third-party, donor-derived VST cells have been investigated in allogeneic SCT and appear to induce reduced levels of GvHD, presumably due to their restricted, virus-specific, repertoire, and memory T cell phenotype. Examples include allogeneic EBV-specific T cells transduced to express CAR19 (Curran et al. 2011) and anti-CD30 CAR (Savoldo 2007).

Alternative Immune Effector Cells

Immune effector cells not associated with induction of GvHD, including NK cells modified via lentiviral transduction to express CAR 19, exhibited early phase efficacy in CLL (Liu et al. 2020). Similarly, iNKT or γδT cells may have advantages against solid tumours, but clinical experience is still limited (Gentles et al. 2015). Engineering of CAR macrophages with antitumour properties has also been described recently (Klichinsky et al. 2020).

Strategies to Avoid Host-Mediated Rejection of Allogeneic Immune Cells

Beyond partial HLA matching of third-party donor cell banks, there are two main strategies to address the risk of host-mediated rejection.

Resistance to Lymphodepletion and Immunosuppression

CAR-T cells have been genome edited to become resistant to an anti-CD52 monoclonal antibody through disruption of CD52 (Benjamin et al. 2020). This approach has the advantage of suppressing all CD52+ immune cells that can mediate rejection, such as T, B, and NK cells, although prolonged immunosuppression is associated with a higher risk of serious virus reactivation. Engineering strategies have also been used to confer resistance to calcineurin inhibitors. Manufacturing steps can be multiplexed alongside editing of the TCR locus during electroporation or added to the vector design and incorporated into transduction steps.

Removal of HLA for Evading Host Immunity

Removal of HLA class I molecules on the cell surface to avoid $CD8^+$ T cell-mediated rejection can be achieved by disrupting the common beta 2-microglobulin gene. This approach is currently being investigated via multiplexed editing of CAR19 T cells (CRISPR Tx). In theory, the complete absence of HLA class I molecules may increase NK-mediated rejection through 'missing self' responses, and in modelling, this can be prevented by the expression of nonpolymorphic HLA molecules, such as HLA-E. Rejection through recognition of HLA class II on activated T cells may be addressed by disruption of critical transcription factors, such as *CIITA* and *RFXANK* (Depil et al. 2020).

Manufacturing Aspects of 'Off-the-Shelf' CARs

The majority of 'off-the-shelf' T cell therapies have utilized healthy donor peripheral blood mononuclear cells (MNCs) acquired via steady-state leukapheresis, although alternative sources, including whole blood and umbilical cord blood, may be suitable. In the future, immune effector cells may also be derived from induced pluripotent stem cells (iPSCs). Theoretically, a master iPSC cell line has an unlimited capability to self-renew and can be banked and used indefinitely. In general, manipulations must be performed in a clean room setting under GMP conditions with suitable licencing and regulatory approvals. Most cell gene transfer and genome engineering strategies require cells to be actively in mitosis to ensure open chromatin and accessible DNA, and activation steps are crucial early in the manufacturing process. Closed system culture and expansion is now routine, with automation reducing labour intensive aspects. High-quality viral vector preparations and improved electroporation steps for genome editing and supplies of stabilized mRNA have been critical. Cryopreservation in convenient dose formulations and efficient cold chain shipping and storage is an essential component of premanufactured 'off-the-shelf' therapies.

Key Points
- Off-the-shelf allogeneic CAR-T cells devoid of significant GvHD potential can be manufactured.
- αβTCR-deleted CAR-T cells and CAR NK cells have successfully entered the early clinical trial phase.
- Several strategies have been developed to avoid host-mediated rejection of allogeneic effector cells.

References

Benjamin R, et al. Genome-edited, donor-derived allogeneic anti-CD19 chimeric antigen receptor T cells in paediatric and adult B-cell acute lymphoblastic leukaemia: results of two phase 1 studies. Lancet. 2020;396(10266):1885–94.

Bunse M, et al. RNAi-mediated TCR knockdown prevents autoimmunity in mice caused by mixed TCR dimers following TCR gene transfer. Mol Ther. 2014;22(11):1983–91.

Curran KJ, et al. Validation of donor derived virus specific T-lymphocytes genetically modified to target the CD19 antigen for the treatment of relapsed leukemia. Mol Ther. 2011;19:S90.

Depil S, et al. 'Off-the-shelf' allogeneic CAR-T cells: development and challenges. Nat Rev Drug Discov. 2020;19(3):185–99.

Gentles AJ, et al. The prognostic landscape of genes and infiltrating immune cells across human cancers. Nat Med. 2015;21(8):938–45.

Gilham DE, et al. TCR inhibitory molecule as a promising allogeneic NKG2D CAR-T cell approach. J Clin Oncol. 2018;36(15_suppl):e15042–2.

Kamiya T, et al. A novel method to generate T-cell receptor-deficient chimeric antigen receptor T cells. Blood Adv. 2018;2(5):517–28.

Klichinsky M, et al. Human chimeric antigen receptor macrophages for cancer immunotherapy. Nat Biotechnol. 2020;38(8):947–53.

Liu E, et al. Use of CAR-transduced natural killer cells in CD19-positive lymphoid tumors. N Engl J Med. 2020;382(6):545–53.

Qasim W, et al. Molecular remission of infant B-ALL after infusion of universal TALEN gene-edited CAR-T cells. Sci Transl Med. 2017;9(374):eaaj2013.

Savoldo B. Blood. 2007;110(7):2620–30. https://doi.org/10.1182/blood-2006-11-059139.

Part III

Clinical Indications for CAR-T Cells

Paediatric Acute Lymphoblastic Leukaemia (ALL)

10

Peter Bader, Franco Locatelli, and Christina Peters

Acute lymphoblastic leukaemia (ALL) is the most frequent malignant disease in childhood and adolescence, with an annual incidence of approximately 3–4 cases per 100,000 children under 15 years of age. Multimodal chemotherapy forms the base of current ALL treatment. Based on excellent national and international collaboration in consecutive prospective, randomized clinical trials, the prognosis of childhood ALL has significantly improved over time. Currently, up to 90% of all paediatric patients with ALL will survive.

However, 15–20% of ALL patients eventually develop disease relapse. Of these patients, 60–80% will achieve a second complete remission (CR) with intensive chemotherapy regimens. Despite this high probability of obtaining a second CR, patients with early bone marrow relapse (namely those occurring within 30 months from diagnosis) have a poor prognosis even if allogeneic stem cell transplantation (allo-SCT) is used as consolidation therapy (Locatelli et al. 2012). According to data from the Berlin-Frankfurt-Münster Group (BFM), patients can be grouped (S1, S2, S3, and S4) according to the site of relapse, immune phenotype, and the time interval between diagnosis and relapse. In S3 and S4 patients, prognosis is worse compared to S1/S2 children, with survival rates of only 25%–30% in the whole

P. Bader (✉)
Division for Stem Cell Transplantation, Immunology and Intensive Care Medicine, Department for Children and Adolescents, University Hospital Frankfurt, Goethe University, Frankfurt, Germany
e-mail: peter.bader@kgu.de

F. Locatelli
Department of Pediatric Hematology/Oncology and Cell and Gene Therapy, IRCCS Bambino Gesù Children's Hospital, Rome, Italy
e-mail: franco.locatelli@opbg.net

C. Peters
Department of Pediatrics, St. Anna Children's Hospital, Medical University of Vienna, Vienna, Austria
e-mail: christina.peters@stanna.at

© The Author(s) 2022
N. Kröger et al. (eds.), *The EBMT/EHA CAR-T Cell Handbook*,
https://doi.org/10.1007/978-3-030-94353-0_10

cohort of patients (von Stackelberg et al. 2011) and most recently 65% and 69% in patients who achieved remission and could receive a transplant from a matched donor (Peters et al. 2021).

In high-risk patients in CR 1 or in relapsed patients with low-risk profiles (CR2, S2), conventional chemotherapy followed by allo-SCT can cure up to 80% of patients (Peters et al. 2015, 2021). In contrast, in patients who relapse after allo-SCT, long-term survival is unlikely, and only 15% of these patients will survive the disease (Kuhlen et al. 2018). Thus far, long-term survival is only possible through a second allo-SCT if patients can obtain an additional CR and are fit enough to receive a second transplant. Second allo-SCT carries a considerable rate of toxicity and mortality, and treatment lasts approximately 6–8 months; finally, approximately 30% of these patients survive (Yaniv et al. 2018).

Thus, there is an unmet medical need among children and adolescents who have the following conditions:

- Primary refractory ALL,
- Treatment refractory relapsed ALL,
- A second relapse of their ALL, or
- Patients who relapse after allogeneic SCT and
- Patients with very high-risk ALL who should undergo allo-SCT but are not eligible for the procedure for medical reasons.

Consequently, with the introduction of CD-19-directed CAR-T cell therapies, these patients are candidates for clinical studies and finally for licencing trials of different CAR-T cell products (Maude et al. 2018). For this patient group up to the age of 25 years, one CAR-T cell product is currently approved by the FDA and EMA. Children, adolescents, and young adults belonging to one of the abovementioned patient groups have an indication for treatment with CAR-T cell therapies. Whether these are the right candidates who benefit most from the novel treatment options remains to be demonstrated. Prospective studies are planned, and a few have already begun to investigate whether the best benefit of CAR-T cell treatment can be obtained if patients were treated early in the course of the disease.

Key Points
- Patients with ALL in the second relapse, with refractory disease or who relapse after allo-SCT may be considered for CD19 CAR-T cell therapy.
- Effective lymphodepleting chemotherapy is needed to allow expansion of CAR-T cells.
- The level of measurable residual disease (MRD) seems to be correlated with response and durable remission.

References

Kuhlen M, Willasch AM, Dalle JH, Wachowiak J, Yaniv I, Ifversen M, Sedlacek P, Guengoer T, Lang P, Bader P, Sufliarska S, Balduzzi A, Strahm B, von Luettichau I, Hoell JI, Borkhardt A, Klingebiel T, Schrappe M, von Stackelberg A, Glogova E, Poetschger U, Meisel R, Peters C. Outcome of relapse after allogeneic HSCT in children with ALL enrolled in the ALL-SCT 2003/2007 trial. Br J Haematol. 2018;180(1):82–9. Epub 2017 Nov 28. https://doi.org/10.1111/bjh.14965.

Locatelli F, Schrappe M, Bernardo ME, Rutella S. How I treat relapsed childhood acute lympho-blastic leukemia. Blood. 2012;120(14):2807–16. Epub 2012 Aug 15. https://doi.org/10.1182/blood-2012-02-265884.

Maude SL, Laetsch TW, Buechner J, Rives S, Boyer M, Bittencourt H, Bader P, Verneris MR, Stefanski HE, Myers GD, Qayed M, De Moerloose B, Hiramatsu H, Schlis K, Davis KL, Martin PL, Nemecek ER, Yanik GA, Peters C, Baruchel A, Boissel N, Mechinaud F, Balduzzi A, Krueger J, June CH, Levine BL, Wood P, Taran T, Leung M, Mueller KT, Zhang Y, Sen K, Lebwohl D, Pulsipher MA, Grupp SA. Tisagenlecleucel in children and young adults with B-cell lymphoblastic leukemia. N Engl J Med. 2018;378(5):439–48. PMID: 29385370; PMCID: PMC5996391. https://doi.org/10.1056/NEJMoa1709866.

Peters C, Schrappe M, von Stackelberg A, Schrauder A, Bader P, Ebell W, Lang P, Sykora KW, Schrum J, Kremens B, Ehlert K, Albert MH, Meisel R, Matthes-Martin S, Gungor T, Holter W, Strahm B, Gruhn B, Schulz A, Woessmann W, Poetschger U, Zimmermann M, Klingebiel T. Stem-cell transplantation in children with acute lymphoblastic leukemia: a prospective international multicenter trial comparing sibling donors with matched unrelated donors-the ALL-SCT-BFM-2003 trial. J Clin Oncol. 2015;33(11):1265–74. Epub 2015 Mar 9. https://doi.org/10.1200/JCO.2014.58.9747.

Peters C, Dalle JH, Locatelli F, Poetschger U, Sedlacek P, Buechner J, Shaw PJ, Staciuk R, Ifversen M, Pichler H, Vettenranta K, Svec P, Aleinikova O, Stein J, Güngör T, Toporski J, Truong TH, Diaz-de-Heredia C, Bierings M, Ariffin H, Essa M, Burkhardt B, Schultz K, Meisel R, Lankester A, Ansari M, Schrappe M, IBFM Study Group, von Stackelberg A, IntReALL Study Group, Balduzzi A, I-BFM SCT Study Group, Corbacioglu S, EBMT Paediatric Diseases Working Party, Bader P. Total body irradiation or chemotherapy conditioning in childhood ALL: a mul-tinational, randomized, noninferiority phase III study. J Clin Oncol. 2021;39(4):295–307. Epub 2020 Dec 17. https://doi.org/10.1200/JCO.20.02529.

von Stackelberg A, Völzke E, Kühl JS, Seeger K, Schrauder A, Escherich G, Henze G, Tallen G, ALL-REZ BFM Study Group. Outcome of children and adolescents with relapsed acute lym-phoblastic leukaemia and non-response to salvage protocol therapy: a retrospective analysis of the ALL-REZ BFM Study Group. Eur J Cancer. 2011;47(1):90–7. Epub 2010 Oct 20. https://doi.org/10.1016/j.ejca.2010.09.020.

Yaniv I, Krauss AC, Beohou E, Dalissier A, Corbacioglu S, Zecca M, Afanasyev BV, Berger M, Diaz MA, Kalwak K, Sedlacek P, Varotto S, Peters C, Bader P. Second hematopoietic stem cell transplantation for post-transplantation relapsed acute leukemia in children: a retrospective EBMT-PDWP study. Biol Blood Marrow Transplant. 2018;24(8):1629–42. Epub 2018 Mar 13.

Adult Acute Lymphoblastic Leukaemia

11

Elad Jacoby, Nicola Gökbuget, and Arnon Nagler

ALL is a malignancy of lymphoid progenitor cells, with a bimodal incidence, peaking in early childhood and in older age. In children, ALL tends to have an excellent prognosis, with more than 85% of patients achieving long-term survival. The outcome of younger adults has improved considerably as well. However, overall survival decreases with age (Dores et al. 2012), partially due to the different genetic background of adult ALL, with a higher proportion of Philadelphia chromosome-positive (Ph+) ALL and Ph-like and KMT2A rearrangements in comparison to childhood ALL (Iacobucci and Mullighan 2017). The introduction of paediatric-inspired regimens has improved outcomes in adults, but these regimens are less tolerated in older patients (Curran and Stock 2015).

The standard upfront therapy for ALL includes corticosteroids, multiagent chemotherapy, antimetabolite therapy, and intrathecal therapy. Following induction, consolidation and maintenance therapy are initiated. In high-risk cases, allogeneic haematopoietic stem-cell transplantation (allo-HSCT) is considered during the first remission. Adults with relapsed ALL have a poor chance of achieving remission with chemotherapy (Frey and Luger 2015). Novel agents, such as inotuzumab ozogamicin, an antibody–drug conjugate targeting CD22, and blinatumomab, a bispecific engager targeting CD19 and CD3, improve remission rates, but overall survival remains poor (Kantarjian et al. 2016, 2017). Relapse therapy is usually followed by allo-HSCT if not performed earlier. ALL cases refractory to two or more lines of therapy can be considered for CAR-T cell therapy.

E. Jacoby · A. Nagler (✉)
Sheba Medical Center, Tel Aviv University, Ramat Gan, Israel
e-mail: Elad.Jacoby@sheba.health.gov.il; Arnon.Nagler@sheba.health.gov.il

N. Gökbuget
Department of Haematology/Oncology, Goethe University,
Frankfurt am Main, Hessen, Germany
e-mail: goekbuget@em.uni-frankfurt.de

© The Author(s) 2022
N. Kröger et al. (eds.), *The EBMT/EHA CAR-T Cell Handbook*,
https://doi.org/10.1007/978-3-030-94353-0_11

CAR-T Cell Therapy for Adult ALL

Currently, in 2021, no regulatory agency has approved a CAR-T cell product for adult ALL patients above 25 years of age. Young adults aged 18–25 were included in the pivotal ELIANA study and are eligible for tisagenlecleucel (Maude et al. 2018). Other single-institutional studies also included young adults in a paediatric-focused study. Only a few groups have reported clinical trials in adults with ALL (Table 11.1). Most trials include small patient numbers, usually younger adults, and may represent selected patient populations. Remission rates across trials are high, with more than 70% of patients achieving complete remission, regardless of cytogenetic background, prior therapies and age. Occasionally, response rates are reported as intent-to-treat, referring to all included patients in contrast to only those receiving CAR-T cell therapy.

Toxicity has been a significant issue in all trials, and fractionation of the dose by administration of a partial dose on Day 0 and the remainder after several days was shown to be safer (Frey et al. 2019; Park et al. 2018). Several groups also administered lower doses to patients with a high disease burden to prevent toxicity (Roddie et al. 2020). Alternative approaches to enhance safety include earlier administration of tocilizumab and low-dose steroids (Gardner et al. 2019; Kadauke et al. 2021; Liu et al. 2020). Using a novel low affinity CD19 CAR-T cell was also associated with lower toxicity (Ghorashian et al. 2019; Roddie et al. 2020).

The prognostic factors that are associated with higher remission rates and better outcome in adult ALL include lower disease burden, as assessed by the blast count in bone marrow; lower LDH; and higher platelet count prior to lymphodepletion (Hay et al. 2019; Park et al. 2018). Due to the time delay between the detection of relapse and infusion of CAR-T cells, in many cases, it is necessary to deliver bridging therapy. The optimal regimens need to be defined.

Assessing the leukaemia burden before CAR-T-infusion and after potential bridging therapies is recommended because the outcome of patients with a high disease burden is inferior to that of those without persistent disease or minimal residual disease (MRD) only. The results may be inferior in ALL patients previously treated with blinatumomab (Pillai et al. 2019), although this may represent a selection of more resistant patients. TP53 mutations were associated with a worse outcome. Additionally, conditioning with fludarabine and cyclophosphamide was superior to cyclophosphamide alone in adults, similar to findings in children.

Many trials report MRD status determined by flow cytometry post CAR-T cell therapy, showing that almost all remissions are (based on flow-cytometry) MRD negative. Molecular detection of MRD via PCR or next-generation sequencing (NGS) is more sensitive, and NGS-MRD negativity after CAR-T cells has been shown to be associated with an improved long-term outcome (Hay et al. 2019).

Table 11.1 Clinical trials reporting the outcome of adult ALL treated with CAR-T cells

Group	n	LD	Construct	Dose	CR (%)	MRD neg of CR	Consolidative therapy	Comments
U. Penn (Frey et al.)	35	Cy (300 × 6, $n = 25$), Flu/Cy ($n = 5$), other ($n = 3$), none ($n = 2$)	FMC63-41BBz	5×10^8 single/fractionated	24 (69)	100% (flow)	9 HSCT, 15 none	2 y OS 47%; fractionation of dose is safer
FHCRC (Hay et al.)	53	Cyclophosphamide ($n = 11$) vs. flu/cy ($n = 42$)	FMC63-41BBz at CD4:CD8 prespecified ratios	2×10^5/kg ($n = 33$), 2×10^6/kg ($n = 20$)	45 (85)	100% (flow), 71% (20/28 NGS)	18 HSCT, 27 none	Low LDH and high platelet levels pre-LD improve outcome; median OS 20 months in responders
MSKCC (Park et al.)	53	Cyclophosphamide (3 g/m², $n = 43$), Flu/Cy ($n = 10$)	MSKCC-28z	$1–3 \times 10^6$/kg	44 (83%)	72% (32 of 44)	17 HSCT, 26 none, 1 other	Median survival 12.9 months
Beijing (Dai et al.)	6	Flu/Cy	CD19/22 (m971/FMC63)-41BBz	$1.7–3 \times 10^6$/kg	6 (100)	100%		3 relapsed, short follow-up time
UCL AUTO1 (Roddie et al.)	19	Flu/Cy	CAT-41BBz	$10–100 \times 10^6$	16 (84)	100%	2 HSCT, 14 none	
Lu Daopei (Zhang et al.)	110 (39 adults)	Flu/Cy	CD19-28z ($n = 21$), CD19-41BBz ($n = 89$)	$1–10 \times 10^6$/kg	102 (92)	94%	75 HSCT, 27 none	Worse outcome with TP53 mutations

Consolidation After CAR-T Cell Therapy

Despite durable CAR-T cells being applied as definitive therapy for relapsed ALL in children, adult data are controversial. Outcomes were not improved by allo-HSCT in patients treated with CD28-based CAR-T cells, which have short-term persistence (Park et al. 2018). In contrast, adults treated with CLT019 (Frey et al. 2019) had better outcomes if transplanted during CR after CAR-T cell therapy. Several centres recommend allo-HSCT for adult ALL patients following CAR-T cell therapy even in the presence of MRD-negative remission (Hay et al. 2019; Zhang et al. 2020; Zhao et al. 2020). Patients with molecular MRD positivity following CAR-T cell therapy, patients with rapid loss of CAR-T cells, and patients who have not received a previous HSCT are candidates for consolidative HSCT (Jacoby 2019; Jiang et al. 2020).

Relapse After CAR-T Cell Therapy

Relapse after CAR-T cell therapy occurs in 30–50% of patients. In instances of durable CAR-T cells, there is a higher probability that relapsed ALL will not express CD19, occurring in up to 40% of cases. If CAR-T cells are lost early, CD19 expression may be preserved. A second dose of CAR-T cells led to rare responses in patients with ALL who relapsed after CAR-T cell therapy or were refractory to this treatment (Gauthier et al. 2020). Other therapies, such as novel antibody-based or CAR-T cells targeting other antigens, are optional.

> **Key Points**
> - No CAR-T cell product is approved for patients with ALL older than 25 years.
> - Clinical trial data for adult ALL are limited.
> - CAR-T cells appear to me more effective and tolerated better if used in the MRD setting of ALL.
> - The use of consolidative HSCT after CAR-T cells in adults is still a matter of debate.

References

Curran E, Stock W. How I treat acute lymphoblastic leukemia in older adolescents and young adults. Blood. 2015;125:3702–10. https://doi.org/10.1182/blood-2014-11-551481.

Dores GM, Devesa SS, Curtis RE, Linet MS, Morton LM. Acute leukemia incidence and patient survival among children and adults in the United States, 2001–2007. Blood. 2012;119:34–43. https://doi.org/10.1182/blood-2011-04-347872.

Frey NV, Luger SM. How I treat adults with relapsed or refractory Philadelphia chromosome-negative acute lymphoblastic leukemia. Blood. 2015;126:589–96. https://doi.org/10.1182/blood-2014-09-551937.

Frey NV, Shaw PA, Hexner EO, Pequignot E, Gill S, Luger SM, et al. Optimizing chimeric antigen receptor T-cell therapy for adults with acute lymphoblastic leukemia. J Clin Oncol. 2019;38:415–22.

Gardner RA, Ceppi F, Rivers J, Annesley C, Summers C, Taraseviciute A, et al. Preemptive mitigation of CD19 CAR-T cell cytokine release syndrome without attenuation of antileukemic efficacy. Blood. 2019;134:2149–58. https://doi.org/10.1182/blood.2019001463.

Gauthier J, Bezerra ED, Hirayama AV, Fiorenza S, Sheih A, Chou CK, et al. Factors associated with outcomes after a second CD19-targeted CAR-T cell infusion for refractory B cell malignancies. Blood. 2020;137:323–35. https://doi.org/10.1182/blood.2020006770.

Ghorashian S, Kramer AM, Onuoha S, Wright G, Bartram J, Richardson R, et al. Enhanced CAR-T cell expansion and prolonged persistence in pediatric patients with ALL treated with a low-affinity CD19 CAR. Nat Med. 2019;25(9):1408–14. https://doi.org/10.1038/s41591-019-0549-5.

Hay KA, Gauthier J, Hirayama AV, Voutsinas JM, Wu Q, Li D, et al. Factors associated with durable EFS in adult B-cell ALL patients achieving MRD-negative CR after CD19 CAR-T cells. Blood. 2019;133:1652–63. https://doi.org/10.1182/blood-2018-11-883710.

Iacobucci I, Mullighan CG. Genetic basis of acute lymphoblastic leukemia. J Clin Oncol. 2017;35:975–83. https://doi.org/10.1200/JCO.2016.70.7836.

Jacoby E. The role of allogeneic HSCT after CAR-T cells for acute lymphoblastic leukemia. Bone Marrow Transplant. 2019;54:810–4. https://doi.org/10.1038/s41409-019-0604-3.

Jiang H, Hu Y, Mei H. Consolidative allogeneic hematopoietic stem cell transplantation after chimeric antigen receptor T-cell therapy for relapsed/refractory B-cell acute lymphoblastic leukemia: who? when? why? Biomark Res. 2020;8:66. https://doi.org/10.1186/s40364-020-00247-8.

Kadauke S, Myers RM, Li Y, Aplenc R, Baniewicz D, Barrett DM, et al. Risk-adapted preemptive tocilizumab to prevent severe cytokine release syndrome after CTL019 for pediatric B-cell acute lymphoblastic leukemia: a prospective clinical trial. J Clin Oncol. 2021;39(8):920–30. https://doi.org/10.1200/jco.20.02477.

Kantarjian HM, DeAngelo DJ, Stelljes M, Martinelli G, Liedtke M, Stock W, et al. Inotuzumab Ozogamicin versus standard therapy for acute lymphoblastic leukemia. N Engl J Med. 2016;375:740–53. https://doi.org/10.1056/NEJMoa1509277.

Kantarjian H, Stein A, Gökbuget N, Fielding AK, Schuh AC, Ribera J-M, et al. Blinatumomab versus chemotherapy for advanced acute lymphoblastic leukemia. N Engl J Med. 2017;376:836–47. https://doi.org/10.1056/NEJMoa1609783.

Liu S, Deng B, Yin Z, Pan J, Lin Y, Ling Z, et al. Corticosteroids do not influence the efficacy and kinetics of CAR-T cells for B-cell acute lymphoblastic leukemia. Blood Cancer J. 2020;10:20–3. https://doi.org/10.1038/s41408-020-0280-y.

Maude SL, Latesch T, Buechner J, Rives S, Boyer M, Bittencourt H, et al. Tisagenlecleucel in children and young adults with B-cell lymphoblastic leukemia. N Engl J Med. 2018;378:439–48. https://doi.org/10.1056/NEJMoa1709866.

Park JH, Rivière I, Gonen M, Wang X, Sénéchal B, Curran KJ, et al. Long-term follow-up of CD19 CAR-therapy in acute lymphoblastic leukemia. N Engl J Med. 2018;378:449–59. https://doi.org/10.1056/NEJMoa1709919.

Pillai V, Muralidharan K, Meng W, Bagashev A, Oldridge DA, Rosenthal J, et al. CAR-T cell therapy is effective for CD19-dim B-lymphoblastic leukemia but is impacted by prior blinatumomab therapy. Blood Adv. 2019;3:3539–49. https://doi.org/10.1182/bloodadvances.2019000692.

Roddie C, O'Reilly MA, Marzolini MAV, Wood L, Dias J, Cadinanos Garai A, et al. ALLCAR19: updated data using AUTO1, a novel fast-off rate CD19 CAR in relapsed/refractory B-cell acute lymphoblastic Leukaemia and other B-cell malignancies. Blood. 2020;136:3–4. https://doi.org/10.1182/blood-2020-137768.

Zhang X, Lu XA, Yang J, Zhang G, Li J, Song L, et al. Efficacy and safety of anti-CD19 CAR-T cell therapy in 110 patients with B-cell acute lymphoblastic leukemia with high-risk features. Blood Adv. 2020;4:2325–38. https://doi.org/10.1182/bloodadvances.2020001466.

Zhao H, Wei J, Wei G, Luo Y, Shi J, Cui Q, et al. Pre-transplant MRD negativity predicts favorable outcomes of CAR-T therapy followed by haploidentical HSCT for relapsed/refractory acute lymphoblastic leukemia: a multi-center retrospective study. J Hematol Oncol. 2020;13:1–13. https://doi.org/10.1186/s13045-020-00873-7.

Diffuse Large B Cell Lymphoma and Primary Mediastinal Lymphoma

12

Bertram Glass and Marie José Kersten

The outcome of patients with large B cell lymphoma (LBCL) who did not respond to a classical immunochemotherapy regimen at any time or relapsed within 1 year following chemoimmunotherapy is poor. The Scholar-One-Study showed long-term event-free survival for less than 20% of these patients (Crump et al. 2017). The introduction of chimeric antigen receptor T cell therapy (CAR-T) is a substantial advancement for these patients, offering long-term remission and a curative prospect for 30 to 40% of patients (summarized in Table 12.1), (Abramson et al. 2020; Neelapu et al. 2017; Schuster et al. 2019b). To date, in Europe, two products (axicabtagene ciloleucel and tisagenlecleucel) have been licenced by the European Medical Agency, and a third product (lisocabtagene maraleucel) will become available in 2022. All these products are licenced for patients who have failed at least two prior lines of systemic therapy. This initially defines, however broad, a range of possible situations in which the application of CART is indicated. The following considerations may help to further define the patient population that should be offered CAR-T cells as the next line of treatment. Recently the results of three randomized phase III clinical studies comparing CD19-CART with standard of Care in transplant eligible patients were reported. The BELINDA-Trial using Tisa-cel did not reach its primary endpoint EFS (Bishop et al. 2021). Two of the studies, ZUMA-7 using the construct Axi-cel and TRANSFORM using Liso-cel were positive for their primary endpoint EFS as well as for the key secondary endpoints PFS and ORR (Kamdar et al. 2021; Locke et al. 2021). In both studies a strong numerical

B. Glass
Clinic for Haematology, Oncology, Tumour Immunology, and Palliative Care, Helios Klinikum Berlin-Buch, Berlin, Germany
e-mail: Bertram.Glass@helios-gesundheit.de

M. J. Kersten (✉)
Department of Hematology, Amsterdam University Medical Centers, University of Amsterdam, Amsterdam, The Netherlands
e-mail: m.j.kersten@amsterdamumc.nl

Table 12.1 Results of pivotal trials of anti-CD19 CAR-T cell therapy

References	Axi-cel Zuma1	Tisa-cel Juliet	Liso-cel Transcend
n (pts infused vs. apheresed)	101/111 (91%)	115/167 (69%)	294/344 (85%)[a]
Age	58 (23–76)	56 (22–76)	63 (18–86)
Prior lines of therapy (median)	3 (1–8)	2 (1–6)	3 (1–8)
Patients refractory (%)	78 (77%)	61 (55%)	181 (67%)
Bridging therapy (%)	0	92	59
ORR (%)	82	52	73
CR (%)	54	32	53
PFS (%)	41	31	44 (1 year)
TRM (%)	4	0	3

[a]25 patients received a non-conforming product

trend towards a positive result regarding OS was observed with Hazard ratios of 0.72 and 0.51, respectively. TRANSFORM had a short median observation time so the results regarding OS were immature. In both studies showed significant advantages in quality of life for CART therapy over ASCT. Anti-CD19 CART therapy with one of these compounds should be considered standard of care in transplant-eligible patients as second line therapy in R/R LBCL.

Patient Population to Consider: Lymphoma-Specific Aspects

Treatment History

Depending on clinical risk factors, between 5 and 50% of LBCL patients may fail standard first-line immunochemotherapy (Coiffier et al. 2010; Cunningham et al. 2013; Pfreundschuh et al. 2011; Schmitz et al. 2012). Overall, 30–40% of patients will need salvage treatment. Patients eligible for high-dose chemotherapy currently receive a platinum-containing salvage protocol, followed by high-dose chemotherapy and autologous stem cell transplantation (autoSCT). In short, the remission rate varies between 35 and 50%, and with another approximately 50% failure rate after autoSCT, the overall long-term event-free survival rate is in the range of 25%. Thus, approximately 75% of younger patients with relapsed/refractory aggressive B cell lymphoma are theoretically eligible for CAR-T cell therapy. *All young, fit patients without remission after salvage therapy in second-line situations should be considered for CAR-T cell therapy.*

Elderly patients with relapsed or refractory LBCL have poor results with second-line therapy. An analysis of the secondary overall survival of patients in a large randomized first-line study revealed that patients with primary refractory disease never achieved long-term remission, and the median overall survival was less than 6 months (Glass et al. 2017). In 20–30% of patients, induction of remission is possible with platinum- or bendamustine-containing regimens, such as

R-gemcitabine-oxaliplatin; however, due to the lack of effective consolidative therapy, the long-term outcome was poor in all series (Dhanapal et al. 2017; Franch-Sarto et al. 2019). In the three pivotal CD19 CAR-T trials, 23–42% of patients were ≥65 years old, and there are currently no indications that the efficacy of CAR-T cells in terms of remission rate and progression-free survival is inferior for elderly patients (Neelapu, Schuster, Abramson). In a real-world series, the percentage of elderly patients was higher, and there was some evidence of increased toxicity, especially neurotoxicity, but the efficacy appeared to be at last equal (Pasquini CIBMTR, Nastoupil).

Therefore, the option of CAR-T cell therapy must be discussed for most transplant ineligible but fit patients with relapsed or refractory aggressive B cell lymphoma after 2 prior lines of systemic therapy.

Remission Status and Tumour Bulk Prior to CAR-T Cell Infusion

CAR-T cells have been evaluated in patients with refractory and early relapsed disease. In pivotal studies of the three licenced CAR-T products, the fraction of refractory patients varied between 52 and 79%. Being refractory to the last line of chemotherapy was not a significant prognostic factor in these studies. Therefore, in contrast to autologous or allogeneic SCT, being in remission is not a prerequisite for the application of CAR-T therapy. However, pivotal clinical studies and the first real-world evidence reports identify high tumour volume, reflected by the sum of product diameters (SPD) or simply an elevated LDH, prior to lymphodepleting therapy as a significant negative prognostic factor for the ongoing complete response rate or PFS (Nastoupil et al. 2020), with a hazard ratio of 3.0. In addition, patients with rapidly progressing disease often do not respond to attempts at bridging therapy, and the need for systemic bridging therapy is a negative predictor for response and survival.

When discussing the value of CAR-T cell therapy for an individual patient, this parameter—disease control prior to CAR-T cell infusion—must be considered. However, this parameter also has an impact on the results of any alternative treatment, and at which point CAR-T cell therapy cannot achieve long-term remission and should not be offered is still a matter of debate.

Histology

The majority of patients in ZUMA-1, JULIET, and TRANSCEND had DLBCL (76%, 80% and 64%); transformed FL was present in 16–22% of cases, and only a small number of patients with PMBCL (8% in ZUMA-1 and 6% in TRANSCEND) were included. Data on DH/TH lymphoma were not available for all patients. There were no significant differences in response rates or PFS in specific subgroups.

Patient Population to Consider: Patient-Specific Aspects

CAR-T cell therapy can lead to unusual and sometimes severe acute toxicities, with cytokine release syndrome (CRS) and immune effector cell-associated neurotoxicity (ICANS) being the most important. These toxicities typically occur between Day 2 and Day 10 after infusion and may persist for several days to weeks. Treatment-related mortality is a rare event, and in most cases, the toxicity is reversible. Other important side effects include severe neutropenia, which may last for several weeks or months, long-term B cell depletion, and hypogammaglobulinaemia, which is an on-target off-tumour toxicity. Compared to the morbidity and mortality associated with other treatment modalities applied in this situation, such as allogeneic SCT, the impact of CAR-T cell-associated toxicity on the overall outcome is moderate. It has been claimed that the good results of CAR-T therapy in terms of toxicity are due to the strict eligibility criteria of the pivotal studies, but recent analyses of data from real-world application of CAR-T therapy showed that efficacy and toxicity were similar, even if elderly and more comorbid patients were treated (Nastoupil et al. 2020). The risk factors for TRM after CAR-T cell therapy are not well defined, and conclusions from other treatment options might be difficult to transfer to CAR-T cell therapy. The best approximation might be the use of the high-dose chemotherapy comorbidity index and its results for patients undergoing autologous SCT. In such an analysis, the HDT-correlated NRM ranged from 3.3 to 7.7% (Berro et al. 2017) after 1 year, which is in line with what has been observed after CAR-T cell therapy (therapy-related mortality <5%).

Alternative Treatments

In the past, allogeneic stem cell transplantation was the only option for consolidation in chemorefractory patients after additional salvage therapy. Recently, antibody–drug conjugates and bispecific antibodies have shown interesting results in the patient population discussed here. Polatuzumab vedotin, the first drug in these groups, has been licenced in Europe and the USA. Many other drugs may enter the arena in the near future. Integration of CAR-T cell therapy with these new treatment options will be a major task in the future.

- Allogeneic stem cell transplantation

   In the past, alloSCT has mostly been used in patients who relapse after autologous stem cell transplantation, and data have been reported from international registries (Fenske et al. 2016; van Kampen et al. 2011). One prospective clinical trial in patients with high-risk aggressive lymphoma showed a PFS and OS of 39% and 40%, respectively, after 4 years (Glass et al. 2014). Taking the potential bias of indirect comparison of treatment results between studies and registry data into account, it can be grossly stated that in many series of allogeneic stem cell transplantation, the overall results in terms of progression-free survival may be comparable to that of CAR-T therapy; however, the balance between the anti-

Table 12.2 Results of prospective randomized trials of second-line treatment for aggressive B-NHL

Study	Salvage regimen	ORR (%)		PFS/EFS		OS		FU	References
CORAL	R-DHAP	62.8	51[a]	42%	21%[a]	51%	40%[a]	3 years	Gisselbrecht et al. (2010)
	R-ICE	63.5		31%	EFS	47%			
NCIC-CTG LY.12[b]	R-DHAP	44.1		26% EFS		39%		4 years	Crump et al. (2014)
	R-GDP	45.1		26% EFS		39%			
ORCHARD	R-DHAP	42		26%		38%		2 years	van Imhoff et al. (2017)
	O-DHAP	38		24%		41%			

[a]Results in patients receiving rituximab as first-line therapy
[b] The study included 8% of patients with T cell lymphoma; 67% of patients received prior rituximab

lymphoma effect and toxicity is dramatically different from that of CAR-T therapy. Treatment-related mortality and morbidity are dramatically higher after allogeneic stem cell transplantation in any age group of patients. Thus, currently, even in patients eligible for alloSCT, CAR-T cells should be offered first. Allogeneic SCT remains a treatment modality that should be considered in patients failing CART therapy, provided they respond to salvage treatment.

- Antibody drug conjugates

  Polatuzumab vedotin is the first ADC that has been licenced for transplant-ineligible patients with DLBCL after failure of at least one prior therapy. In the pivotal randomized phase II study (Sehn et al. 2020a) and the recently reported expansion cohort (Sehn et al. 2020b), the patient population treated was comparable to the populations in most of the CAR-T cell studies. The best overall response rate was 57.9%, with a CR rate of 52.6%. Some of the responses seem to be ongoing after the end of treatment. With the limited number of patients and the limited observation time, it can be estimated that approximately 15–20% of patients might be in ongoing remission after 2 years. Thus, the potential to serve as a curative treatment is small if it exists at all, and a longer follow-up time and validation in other prospective clinical trials are warranted. ADCs, such as polatuzumab vedotin, might be good candidates for achieving control of the disease prior to CAR-T cell application in a so-called bridging approach. Polatuzumab is licenced in combination with bendamustine, a drug with exceptionally high T cell toxicity. The application of bendamustine should be avoided prior to apheresis of autologous T cells for CAR-T cell production.

- Bispecific antibodies

  A number of bispecific, T cell-engaging antibodies using the CD20 antigen as a lymphoma-specific target and CD3 as a T cell binding site have been reported with very encouraging results (Table 12.2) (Bannerji et al. 2020; Hutchings et al. 2020a,b; Schuster et al. 2019a). The response rates are high for some of the agents, and the toxicity is quite limited. However, the observation time is still short, and data on PFS are not yet available. There is an indication that the DOR of patients achieving CR is particularly good thus far and in the same range as that observed in trials of CAR-T cells. Bispecific antibodies may have the potential to induce long-lasting remissions without further consolidation, but this treatment is often given until progression or toxicity occurs. Once available in routine practice, their differential indication for treatment compared to CAR-T cells will become an important clinical challenge and should preferably be investigated in head-to-head clinical trials.

Key Points
- Patients with LBCL, including transformed FL and PMBCL, should be considered for CD19 CAR-T cell therapy in cases of relapsed/refractory disease after ≥2 lines of systemic therapy.
- There is no upper age limit, but patients should fulfil eligibility criteria in terms of fitness, cardiac function, and other organ functions.
- Patients with high LDH and rapidly progressing disease are less likely to benefit.

References

Abramson JS, Palomba ML, Gordon LI, Lunning MA, Wang M, Arnason J, et al. Lisocabtagene maraleucel for patients with relapsed or refractory large B-cell lymphomas (TRANSCEND NHL 001): a multicentre seamless design study. Lancet. 2020;396:839–52.

Bannerji R, Allan JN, Arnason JE, Brown JR, Advani R, Ansell SM, et al. Odronextamab (REGN1979), a human CD20 x CD3 bispecific antibody, induces durable, complete responses in patients with highly refractory B-cell non-Hodgkin lymphoma, including patients refractory to CAR-T therapy. Blood. 2020;136:42–3.

Berro M, Arbelbide JA, Rivas MM, Basquiera AL, Ferini G, Vitriu A, et al. Hematopoietic cell transplantation-specific comorbidity index predicts morbidity and mortality in autologous stem cell transplantation. Biol Blood Marrow Transplant. 2017;23:1646–50.

Bishop MR, Dickinson M, Purtill D, Barba P, Santoro A, Hamad N, et al. Second-Line tisagenlecleucel or standard care in aggressive B-Cell lymphoma. N Engl J Med. 2021. Dec 14, Online ahead of print.

Coiffier B, Thieblemont C, Van Den Neste E, Lepeu G, Plantier I, Castaigne S, et al. Long-term outcome of patients in the LNH-98.5 trial, the first randomized study comparing rituximab-CHOP to standard CHOP chemotherapy in DLBCL patients: a study by the Groupe d'Etudes des Lymphomes de l'Adulte. Blood. 2010;116:2040–5.

Crump M, Kuruvilla J, Couban S, Macdonald DA, Kukreti V, Kouroukis CT, et al. Randomized comparison of gemcitabine, dexamethasone, and cisplatin versus dexamethasone, cytarabine, and cisplatin chemotherapy before autologous stem-cell transplantation for relapsed and refractory aggressive lymphomas: NCIC-CTG LY.12. J Clin Oncol. 2014;32:3490–6.

Crump M, Neelapu SS, Farooq U, Van Den Neste E, Kuruvilla J, Westin J, et al. Outcomes in refractory diffuse large B-cell lymphoma: results from the international SCHOLAR-1 study. Blood. 2017;130:1800–8.

Cunningham D, Hawkes EA, Jack A, Qian W, Smith P, Mouncey P, et al. Rituximab plus cyclophosphamide, doxorubicin, vincristine, and prednisolone in patients with newly diagnosed diffuse large B-cell non-Hodgkin lymphoma: a phase 3 comparison of dose intensification with 14-day versus 21-day cycles. Lancet. 2013;381:1817–26.

Dhanapal V, Gunasekara M, Lianwea C, Marcus R, De Lord C, Bowcock S, et al. Outcome for patients with relapsed/refractory aggressive lymphoma treated with gemcitabine and oxaliplatin with or without rituximab; a retrospective, multicentre study. Leuk Lymphoma. 2017;58:1–9.

Fenske TS, Ahn KW, Graff TM, DiGilio A, Bashir Q, Kamble RT, et al. Allogeneic transplantation provides durable remission in a subset of DLBCL patients relapsing after autologous transplantation. Br J Haematol. 2016;174:235–48.

Franch-Sarto M, Sorigue M, Lopez L, Moreno M, Ribera JM, Sancho JM. Overall survival in patients with relapsed/refractory high grade B-cell lymphomas treated with gemcitabine, oxaliplatin with or without rituximab. Leuk Lymphoma. 2019;60:3324–6.

Gisselbrecht C, Glass B, Mounier N, Singh GD, Linch DC, Trneny M, et al. Salvage regimens with autologous transplantation for relapsed large B-cell lymphoma in the rituximab era. J Clin Oncol. 2010;28:4184–90.

Glass B, Hasenkamp J, Wulf G, Dreger P, Pfreundschuh M, Gramatzki M, et al. Rituximab after lymphoma-directed conditioning and allogeneic stem-cell transplantation for relapsed and refractory aggressive non-Hodgkin lymphoma (DSHNHL R3): an open-label, randomised, phase 2 trial. Lancet Oncol. 2014;15:757–66.

Glass B, Dohm AJ, Truemper LH, Pfreundschuh M, Bleckmann A, Wulf GG, et al. Refractory or relapsed aggressive B-cell lymphoma failing (R)-CHOP: an analysis of patients treated on the RICOVER-60 trial. Ann Oncol. 2017;28:3058–64.

Hutchings M, Carlo-Stella C, Bachy E, Offner FC, Morschhauser F, Crump M, et al. Glofitamab step-up dosing induces high response rates in patients with hard-to-treat refractory or relapsed non-Hodgkin lymphoma. Blood. 2020a;136:46–8.

Hutchings M, Mous R, Clausen MR, Johnson P, Linton KM, Chamuleau MED, et al. Subcutaneous Epcoritamab induces complete responses with an encouraging safety profile across relapsed/refractory B-cell non-Hodgkin lymphoma subtypes, including patients with prior CAR-T therapy: updated dose escalation data. Blood. 2020b;136:45–6.

van Imhoff GW, McMillan A, Matasar MJ, Radford J, Ardeshna KM, Kuliczkowski K, et al. Ofatumumab versus rituximab salvage chemoimmunotherapy in relapsed or refractory diffuse large B-cell lymphoma: the ORCHARRD Study. J Clin Oncol. 2017;35:544.

Kamdar M, Solomon SR, Arnason JE, Johnston PB, Glass B, Bachanova V, et al. Lisocabtagene Maraleucel (liso-cel), a CD19-Directed Chimeric Antigen Receptor (CAR) T Cell Therapy, Versus Standard of Care (SOC) with Salvage Chemotherapy (CT) Followed By Autologous Stem Cell Transplantation (ASCT) As Second-Line (2L) Treatment in Patients (Pts) with Relapsed or Refractory (R/R) Large B-Cell Lymphoma (LBCL): Results from the Randomized Phase 3 Transform Study. Blood. 2021;138:91–91.

van Kampen RJ, Canals C, Schouten HC, Nagler A, Thomson KJ, Vernant JP, et al. Allogeneic stem-cell transplantation as salvage therapy for patients with diffuse large B-cell non-Hodgkin's lymphoma relapsing after an autologous stem-cell transplantation: an analysis of the European Group for Blood and Marrow Transplantation Registry. J Clin Oncol. 2011;29:1342–8.

Locke FL, Miklos DB, Jacobson CA, Perales MA, Kersten MJ, Oluwole OO, et al. Axicabtagene ciloleucel as second-line therapy for large B-Cell lymphoma. N Engl J Med. 2021. 14 Dec, Online ahead of print.

Nastoupil LJ, Jain MD, Feng L, Spiegel JY, Ghobadi A, Lin Y, et al. Standard-of-care Axicabtagene Ciloleucel for relapsed or refractory large B-cell lymphoma: results from the US Lymphoma CAR-T Consortium. J Clin Oncol. 2020;38:3119–28.

Neelapu SS, Locke FL, Bartlett NL, Lekakis LJ, Miklos DB, Jacobson CA, et al. Axicabtagene Ciloleucel CAR-T cell therapy in refractory large B-cell lymphoma. N Engl J Med. 2017;377:2531–44.

Pfreundschuh M, Kuhnt E, Trumper L, Osterborg A, Trneny M, Shepherd L, et al. CHOP-like chemotherapy with or without rituximab in young patients with good-prognosis diffuse large-B-cell lymphoma: 6-year results of an open-label randomised study of the MabThera International Trial (MInT) Group. Lancet Oncol. 2011;12:1013–22.

Schmitz N, Nickelsen M, Ziepert M, Haenel M, Borchmann P, Schmidt C, et al. Conventional chemotherapy (CHOEP-14) with rituximab or high-dose chemotherapy (MegaCHOEP) with rituximab for young, high-risk patients with aggressive B-cell lymphoma: an open-label, randomised, phase 3 trial (DSHNHL 2002-1). Lancet Oncol. 2012;13:1250.

Schuster SJ, Bartlett NL, Assouline S, Yoon SS, Bosch F, Sehn LH, et al. Mosunetuzumab induces complete remissions in poor prognosis non-Hodgkin lymphoma patients, including those who are resistant to or relapsing after chimeric antigen receptor T-cell (CAR-T) therapies, and is active in treatment through multiple lines. Blood. 2019a;134:6.

Schuster SJ, Bishop MR, Tam CS, Waller EK, Borchmann P, McGuirk JP, et al. Tisagenlecleucel in adult relapsed or refractory diffuse large B-cell lymphoma. N Engl J Med. 2019b;380:45–56.

Sehn LH, Herrera AF, Flowers CR, Kamdar MK, McMillan A, Hertzberg M, et al. Polatuzumab vedotin in relapsed or refractory diffuse large B-cell lymphoma. J Clin Oncol. 2020a;38:155–65.

Sehn LH, Hertzberg M, Opat S, Herrera AF, Assouline SE, Flowers C, et al. Polatuzumab vedotin plus bendamustine and rituximab in relapsed/refractory diffuse large B-cell lymphoma: updated results of a phase Ib/II randomized study and preliminary results of a single-arm extension. Blood. 2020b;136:17–9.

Mantle Cell Lymphoma

13

Noel Milpied and Martin Dreyling

Mantle cell lymphoma is a distinct lymphoma subtype with a widely varying clinical course. Established high-risk biological factors include blastoid cytomorphology, high cell proliferation (Ki-67 > 67%), and *p53* mutations (Aukema et al. 2018). While current first-line approaches are still chemotherapy-based, BTK inhibitors are the preferred targeted approach, especially in early relapse cases (POD24) (Dreyling et al. 2017; Visco et al. 2021). However, cases of relapse/progression under BTK inhibitors display extremely aggressive features with a dismal outcome after conventional regimens (Martin et al. 2016).

Clinical Indications for CAR-T Cells

Following a conditional marketing authorization issued by the EMA in December 2020, Tecartus® (Gilead) is the first autologous anti-CD-19 CAR-T cell therapy that can be administered to patients with mantle cell lymphoma in Europe. Patients deemed eligible for this treatment are those with histologically verified mantle cell lymphoma resistant to or relapsing after two or more lines of treatment, including a Bruton tyrosine kinase (BTK) inhibitor.

This registration is based on the results of recently reported a multicentre phase 2 trial (Wang et al. 2020a). Briefly, 74 patients with a median age of 65 (38–79) were enrolled, and 88% were refractory to or relapsed after BTK inhibitor treatment at any time point. The CAR-T cell product could be manufactured for 71, and 68

N. Milpied
Department of Hematology and Stem Cell Transplantation, Centre Hospitalier Universitaire, Bordeaux, France
e-mail: noel.milpied@chru-bordeaux.fr

M. Dreyling (✉)
Department of Medicine III, LMU Hospital, Munich, Germany
e-mail: martin.dreyling@med.uni-muenchen.de

© The Author(s) 2022
N. Kröger et al. (eds.), *The EBMT/EHA CAR-T Cell Handbook*,
https://doi.org/10.1007/978-3-030-94353-0_13

Table 13.1 Updated response rates (Wang et al. 2020b)

	ORR (%)	CR (%)	PFS (%)		OS (%)	
			12 m	15 m	12 m	15 m
Intent to Tx (74 patients)	85	59				
Prim analysis (60 patients)	93	67	61	59	83	76

received 2×10^6 CAR-T cells/kg on Day 0 after a conditioning regimen consisting of fludarabine (30 mg/m²/day) and cyclophosphamide (500 mg/m²/day) from Day 5 to Day 3. The overall response rate of all 74 patients (intent-to-treat population) was 85%, with a CR rate of 59%. More importantly, after 15 months, 59% of the 60 evaluable patients were still in remission (Wang et al. 2020b) (Table 13.1).

Interestingly, in contrast to conventional strategies, the percentages of patients with an objective response were consistent among key subgroups, including patients with high-risk features (Wang et al. 2020a).

Adverse events were mainly cytopenias ($\geq$ grade 3: 94%) and infections ($\geq$ grade 3: 32%). A total of 26% of the patients had grade 3 or higher cytopenias more than 90 days after the administration of KTE-X19, including neutropenia (in 16% of patients), thrombocytopenia (16%), and anaemia (12%).

These encouraging results have also been confirmed for another CAR-T cell construct (Lisocabtagene Maraleucel; Palomba et al. 2020).

Critical Evaluation

These excellent results were achieved in the context of a prospective study in highly selected patients. Recently similar results have been reported in a "real life setting" (Wang et al. 2021).

In the current algorithm of the approved indication, several other conditions must be fulfilled before implementation of this treatment: careful work-up of the patient, an experienced interdisciplinary team, and a specialized hospital with follow-up resources. In future trials, the benefit–risk ratio of this demanding treatment will be rechallenged in earlier treatment lines.

Key Points
- Patients with relapsed MCL progressing under the BTK inhibitor ibrutinib should be considered for CD19 CAR-T cell therapy.
- Effective lymphodepleting chemotherapy is needed to allow expansion of CAR-T cells.

References

Aukema SM, Hoster E, Rosenwald A, et al. Expression of TP53 is associated with the outcome of MCL independent of MIPI and Ki-67 in trials of the European MCL Network. Blood. 2018;131(4):417–20.

Dreyling M, Campo E, Hermine O, et al. Newly diagnosed and relapsed mantle cell lymphoma: ESMO clinical practice guidelines for diagnosis, treatment and follow-up. Ann Oncol. 2017;28(Suppl_4):iv62–71.

Martin P, Maddocks K, Leonard JP, et al. Postibrutinib outcomes in patients with mantle cell lymphoma. Blood. 2016;127(12):1559–63.

Palomba ML, Gordon LI, Siddiqi T, et al. Safety and preliminary efficacy in patients with relapsed/refractory mantle cell lymphoma receiving Lisocabtagene Maraleucel in TRANSCEND NHL 001. ASH; 2020, #118.

Visco C, Di Rocco A, Evangelista A, et al. Outcomes in first relapsed-refractory younger patients with mantle cell lymphoma: results from the MANTLE-FIRST study. Leukemia. 2021;35(3):787–95.

Wang M, Munoz J, Goy A, et al. KTE-X19 CAR-T cell therapy in relapsed or refractory mantle-cell lymphoma. N Engl J Med. 2020a;382:1331–42.

Wang M, Munoz J, Goy A, et al. One-year follow-up of ZUMA-2, the multicenter, registrational study of KTE-X19 in patients with relapsed/refractory mantle cell lymphoma. ASH; 2020b, #1120.

Wang Y, Jain P, Locke FL, et al. Brexucabtagene autoleucel for relapsed/refractory mantle cell lymphoma: real world experience from the US lymphoma CAR T consortium. ASH 2021, #744.

Chronic Lymphocytic Leukaemia

14

Olivier Tournilhac and Peter Dreger

Clinical Development of CAR-T Cells for CLL

Although chronic lymphocytic leukaemia (CLL) was one of the first two entities in which CAR-T cells were evaluated, it has not yet arrived in the clinical routine. Since the landmark study by Porter et al. (2011), only six CLL-specific clinical trials have been published, altogether comprising no more than 155 patients (Porter et al. 2015; Gill et al. 2018; Turtle et al. 2017; Gauthier et al. 2020; Siddiqi et al. 2020; Wierda et al. 2020; Frey et al. 2020). All six of these studies investigated CD19-directed CAR-T constructs in heavily pretreated patients, mostly having failed BTKi +/− venetoclax therapy. Despite overall response rates of 60–95%, including MRD clearance in a large proportion of patients, the CR rates appear to be relatively low, and only a few durable responses have been reported in patients achieving a CR (Porter et al. 2015; Frey et al. 2020; Cappell et al. 2020). While toxicity includes 5–20% grade 3 cytokine release syndrome and 5–25% grade 3 neurotoxicity and appears manageable, long-term efficacy remains an unresolved issue. CLL-specific efficacy barriers for CD19 CAR-T cells could include a reduced capacity for sustained T cell expansion in extensively pretreated elderly CLL patients (Lemal and Tournilhac 2019), along with impaired T cell motility, impaired T cell mitochondrial fitness, and T cell exhaustion (Bair and Porter 2019). Concurrent use of ibrutinib might reduce the CRS rate and severity (Gauthier et al. 2020; Gill et al. 2018; Wierda et al. 2020) without impairing CAR-T cell expansion.

O. Tournilhac (✉)
Service d'Hematologie Clinique et de Therapie Cellulaire, CHU, Universite Clermont Auvergne, Clermont Ferrand, France
e-mail: otournilhac@chu-clermontferrand.fr

P. Dreger
Department of Medicine V, Hematology, Oncology and Rheumatology, University Hospital Heidelberg, Heidelberg, Germany
e-mail: peter.dreger@med.uni-heidelberg.de

© The Author(s) 2022
N. Kröger et al. (eds.), *The EBMT/EHA CAR-T Cell Handbook*,
https://doi.org/10.1007/978-3-030-94353-0_14

Current Indications for CAR-T Cells in the Treatment Landscape of CLL

In the absence of studies with informative sample sizes and follow-up and without an approved CAR-T cell preparation available, there is currently no indication for CAR-T cells in CLL outside of a clinical trial. However, if a suitable trial is available, CAR-T cells can be proposed as an alternative in patients with high-risk-2 CLL who have a high transplant risk according to the EBMT-ERIC recommendations (Dreger et al. 2018). In patients with a low transplant risk, allogeneic haematopoietic cell transplantation (alloHCT) still appears to be the more promising approach in terms of long-term disease control (Tournilhac et al. 2020; Roeker et al. 2020; Mato et al. 2020). The advent of more effective CAR-T cell therapies for CLL is eagerly awaited and may rapidly change this algorithm.

> - **Currently, there is no standard indication for CAR-T cells in CLL.**
> - **CAR-T cells may be an alternative to alloHCT in high-risk patients in clinical trials.**

Prospective Studies of Autologous Anti-CD19 CAR-T Cell Therapy for CLL

	Porter et al. (2015)	Frey et al. (2020)	Gill et al. (2018)	Turtle et al. (2017)	Gauthier et al. (2020)	Siddiqi et al. (2020)	Wierda et al. (2020)
Patients (n)	14	38	19	24 (5RT)	19 (4RT)	22 (1RT)	19
CAR-T with ibrutinib	CTL019 No	CART-19 No	CTL119 Yes	JCAR014 No	JCAR014 Yes	JCAR017[a] No	JCAR017[a] Yes
Age (years)	66 (51–78)	61 (49–76)	62 (42–76)	61 (40–73)	65 (40–71)	66 (50–80)	60 (50–77)
Previous lines (n)	5 (1–11)	3.5 (2–7)	2 (1–16)	5 (3–9)	5 (1–10)	4 (2–11)	4 (2–11)
Ibrutinib (R/R)	1 (1)	9 (?)	5 (0)	24 (19)	19 (19)	23 (17)	19 (19)
Venetoclax (R/R)	0	1	0	6 (6)	11 (6)	13 (11)	11 (na)
CK (%)	Na	Na	Na	67	74	48	42
TP53 alt. (%)	43	39[b]	58	Del = 58	Del = 74	Mut = 61 Del = 35	Mut = 32 Del = 42
ORR (%)	57	44[b]	71[b]	70	83[b]	82[b]	95
CR (%)	29	28[b]	43[b]	17	22[b]	46[b]	63
MRD(−) BM (%)	29	na	78[b]	50[b]	61[b]	65[b]	79

	Porter et al. (2015)	Frey et al. (2020)	Gill et al. (2018)	Turtle et al. (2017)	Gauthier et al. (2020)	Siddiqi et al. (2020)	Wierda et al. (2020)
CRS (all/ G3) (%)	64/43	63/24	95/16	83/8	74/0	74/9	74/5
NT (all/ G3) (%)	36/7	na/8	26/5	33/25	26/26	39/22	32/16
FU (m)	19 (6–53)	32 (2–75)	19 (8–28)	NA	12 (4–17)	24	10
PFS (m) PFS >24 m (n)	28% @18 m 3	1 m 7	na na	8.5 m na	38% @12 m na	50% @18 m na	na na
NRM (n) cause	1 (infection)	0 /	1 (cardiac)	1 (CRS/ NT)	1 (cardiac)	0 /	0 /

RT Richter transformation, *R/R* relapsed/refractory, *TP53 alt.* TP53 mutation and/or 17p deletion, *CRS* cytokine release syndrome, *NT* neurotoxicity, *allG* all grades, $G \geq 3$ grade ≥ 3, *na* not available, *CK* complex karyotype (≥ 3 abnormalities), *BM* bone marrow, *MRD(−)* BM negative bone marrow minimal residual disease, *NRM* non relapse mortality
[a]Transcend CLL 004 study with lisocabtagene maraleucel
[b]Assessment limited to evaluable patients

Key Points
- Autologous CAR-T cells for CLL have been in development for almost 10 years, with interesting results in poor-risk disease, including patients double refractory to both BTKi and BCL2i.
- However, more data, including clinical trials with a longer follow-up time, are required before adding CAR-T cells to clinical practice.

References

Bair SM, Porter DL. Accelerating chimeric antigen receptor therapy in chronic lymphocytic leukemia: the development and challenges of chimeric antigen receptor T-cell therapy for chronic lymphocytic leukemia. Am J Hematol. 2019;94(Suppl_1):S10–7.

Cappell KM, Sherry RM, Yang JC, et al. Long-term follow-up of anti-CD19 chimeric antigen receptor T-cell therapy. JCO. 2020;38(32):3805–15.

Dreger P, Ghia P, Schetelig J, et al. High-risk chronic lymphocytic leukemia in the era of pathway inhibitors: integrating molecular and cellular therapies. Blood. 2018;132(9):892–902.

Frey NV, Gill S, Hexner EO, et al. Long-term outcomes from a randomized dose optimization study of chimeric antigen receptor modified T cells in relapsed chronic lymphocytic leukemia. JCO. 2020;38:2862.

Gauthier J, Hirayama AV, Purushe J, et al. Feasibility and efficacy of CD19-targeted CAR-T cells with concurrent ibrutinib for CLL after ibrutinib failure. Blood. 2020;135(19):1650–60.

Gill SI, Vides V, Frey NV, et al. Prospective clinical trial of anti-CD19 CAR-T cells in combination with Ibrutinib for the treatment of chronic lymphocytic leukemia shows a high response rate. Blood. 2018;132(Suppl 1):298.

Lemal R, Tournilhac O. State-of-the-art for CAR-T cell therapy for chronic lymphocytic leukemia in 2019. J Immunother Cancer. 2019;7(1):202.

Mato AR, Roeker LE, Jacobs R, et al. Assessment of the efficacy of therapies following Venetoclax discontinuation in CLL reveals BTK inhibition as an effective strategy. Clin Cancer Res. 2020;26(14):3589–96.

Porter DL, Levine BL, Kalos M, Bagg A, June CH. Chimeric antigen receptor–modified T cells in chronic lymphoid leukemia. N Engl J Med. 2011;365(8):725–33.

Porter DL, Hwang W-T, Frey NV, et al. Chimeric antigen receptor T cells persist and induce sustained remissions in relapsed refractory chronic lymphocytic leukemia. Sci Transl Med. 2015;7(303):303ra139.

Roeker LE, Dreger P, Brown JR, et al. Allogeneic stem cell transplantation for chronic lymphocytic leukemia in the era of novel agents. Blood Adv. 2020;4(16):3977–89.

Siddiqi T, Soumerai JD, Dorritie KA, et al. Updated follow-up of patients with relapsed/refractory chronic lymphocytic leukemia/small lymphocytic lymphoma treated with Lisocabtagene Maraleucel in the phase 1 monotherapy cohort of transcend CLL 004, including high-risk and Ibrutinib-treated patients. Blood 2020;136(1):546.

Tournilhac O, Le Garff-Tavernier M, Nguyen Quoc S, et al. Efficacy of minimal residual disease driven immune-intervention after allogeneic hematopoietic stem cell transplantation for high-risk chronic lymphocytic leukemia: results of a prospective multicentric trial. Haematologica. 2020; https://doi.org/10.3324/haematol.2019.239566.

Turtle CJ, Hay KA, Hanafi L-A, et al. Durable molecular remissions in chronic lymphocytic leukemia treated with CD19-specific chimeric antigen receptor-modified T cells after failure of Ibrutinib. J Clin Oncol. 2017;35(26):3010–20.

Wierda W, Dorritie KA, Munoz J, et al. Transcend CLL 004: phase 1 Cohort of Lisocabtagene Maraleucel (liso-cel) in combination with Ibrutinib for patients with Relapsed/Refractory (R/R) chronic lymphocytic leukemia/small lymphocytic lymphoma (CLL/SLL). Blood 2020;136(1):544.

Indolent Lymphomas

15

Franck Morschhauser and Pier Luigi Zinzani

Indolent non-Hodgkin lymphoma (iNHL), including follicular (FL) and marginal zone (MZL) lymphoma, now enjoy durable disease control with first-line immuno-chemotherapy, with a median overall survival (OS) of over 15 years in most series (Kahl and Yang 2016). However, iNHL is still widely considered incurable in most cases, and disease history remains characterized by a relapsing and remitting course, with each remission period shorter than the previous one, and OS and progression-free survival (PFS) decrease with each subsequent line of conventional therapy (Batlevi et al. 2020). Patients with unmet needs include approximately 20% of FL patients who experience disease progression within 24 months (POD24) after initial chemoimmunotherapy (with a 5-year OS of 48% (Casulo et al. 2015)—although it remains unclear how much this worse outcome is driven by misdiagnosed transformed follicular lymphoma (Freeman et al. 2019)); those who fail multiple regimens (5-year PFS of 23%) (Rivas-Delgado et al. 2019), have double refractory disease (Gopal et al. 2017) or experience relapse after autologous stem cell transplantation (ASCT) (Sesques et al. 2020). Although promising results were obtained with an immunomodulatory regimen combining anti-CD20 Moab and lenalidomide (Leonard et al. 2019; Morschhauser et al. 2019), most current approved therapies do not overcome incremental disease resistance, resulting in multiple lines of treatment with cumulative toxicity over a patient's lifetime. The autologous anti-CD19 chimeric antigen receptor T cell (CAR-T) therapies tisa-cel and axi-cel, which are now approved for patients with relapsed/refractory (r/r) large B cell lymphoma (LBCL), have also been tested in iNHL, with promising results.

F. Morschhauser (✉)
Department of Hematology, University of Lille, CHU Lille, ULR 7365 – GRITA – Groupe de Recherche sue les forms injectables et les Technologies Associees, Lille, France
e-mail: f-morschhauser@chru-lille.fr

P. L. Zinzani
Institute of Hematology "L. e A. Seràgnoli" University of Bologna, Bologna, Italy
e-mail: pierluigi.zinzani@unibo.it

83

N. Kröger et al. (eds.), *The EBMT/EHA CAR-T Cell Handbook*,
https://doi.org/10.1007/978-3-030-94353-0_15

The ZUMA-5 phase 2 trial evaluated the efficacy and safety of axi-cel in 146 patients with r/r iNHL (FL: 124; MZL: 22) after at least two lines of therapy (Jacobson et al. 2020). Among the 104 patients available for the efficacy analysis (84 with FL and 20 with MZL), the overall response rate (ORR) was 92%, with 76% of patients obtaining complete remission (CR). In FL patients, the ORR was 94%, with a CR rate of 80%. Response rates were consistent among patients with high-risk features. With a median follow-up of 17.5 months, 64% of FL patients remained in response. The median duration of response (DoR), PFS, and OS were not reached (Gopal et al. 2017). The safety profile was manageable and appeared favourable in patients with FL compared with that previously reported in LBCL (Neelapu et al. 2017; Locke et al. 2019). Grade ≥ 3 adverse events (AEs) occurred in 126 patients (86%), most commonly neutropenia and infection. Fewer instances of any grade (78%) and high-grade (6%) cytokine release syndrome (CRS) were observed in the FL cohort. The onset of CRS was delayed compared with that seen in LBCL. The event was not resolved in only one patient, who ultimately died due to multiorgan failure (Jacobson et al. 2020). Fifty-six percent of patients experienced neurological events (NEs) of any grade; 15% had grade ≥ 3 events. Most NEs (67/70) resolved by the data cut-off time (Jacobson et al. 2020).

The same reliable results were seen with tisa-cel. In the phase 2 ELARA study, 98 adult patients with r/r FL within 6 months after second or later therapy or that relapsed after ASCT were enrolled (Fowler et al. 2020). Ninety-seven patients received tisa-cel, but 52 were evaluable for efficacy. Unlike the ZUMA-5 trial, bridging therapy was allowed, and 43% of patients received it. Thirty-four of 52 patients (65.4%) achieved a CR, with an ORR of 82.7%. With a median follow-up of 9.9 months, 69% of patients were still in response. Median DoR, PFS, and OS were not reached. Of the 97 patients evaluable for safety (median follow-up of 6.6 months), 69% experienced grade ≥ 3 AEs, most commonly neutropenia; 48% of patients had CRS, but none of them experienced a grade ≥ 3 AE. Any grade NEs occurred in 10% of patients; 2% had a grade ≥ 3 NE, and all recovered. No deaths seen were treatment-related (Fowler et al. 2020).

These preliminary data from the ELARA and ZUMA-5 trials suggest that anti-CD19 CAR-T cell treatment is effective in high-risk or extensively treated r/r iNHL, resulting in a high CR and ORR. Although the benefit/risk ratio seems highly favourable in high-risk FL patients, such as young, double refractory, relapse post-ASCT patients or those with POD24, longer follow-up times are needed to better define the potential for cure and the limited long-term toxicities, especially in view of the emergence of highly efficient competitive therapies, such as bispecific antibodies (Bannerji et al. 2020; Hutchings et al. 2020a,b; Assouline et al. 2020). Data remain scarce in MZL. Clearly, phase III randomized trials are mandatory to confirm the role of CAR-T cells in R/R in NHL, especially in POD24 patients.

Key Points
- Anti-CD19 CAR-T cell treatment achieves high CR and ORRs in extensively treated r/r FLs with an acceptable safety profile.
- The response appears durable, but the median follow-up time remains short.
- Data remain scarce in MZL.
- Phase 3 randomized trials are mandatory to confirm the role of CAR-T cells in r/r iNHL, especially in POD24 patients.

References

Assouline SE, Kim WS, Sehn LH, et al. Mosunetuzumab shows promising efficacy in patients with multiply relapsed follicular lymphoma: updated clinical experience from a phase I dose-escalation trial. ASH Congress; 2020, abstract 702.

Bannerji R, Allan JN, Arnason JE, et al. Odronextamab (REGN1979), a human CD20 x CD3 bispecific antibody, induces durable, complete responses in patients with highly refractory B-cell non-Hodgkin lymphoma, including patients refractory to CAR-T therapy ASH Congress; 2020, abstract 400.

Batlevi L, Sha F, Alperovich A, et al. Blood. Cancer J. 2020;10(7):74. https://doi.org/10.1038/s41408-020-00340-z.

Casulo C, Byrtek M, Dawson KL, et al. Early relapse of follicular lymphoma after rituximab plus cyclophosphamide, doxorubicin, vincristine, and prednisone defines patients at high risk for death: an analysis from the National LymphoCare Study. J Clin Oncol. 2015;33(23):2516–22. https://doi.org/10.1200/JCO.2014.59.7534. Epub 2015 Jun 29.

Fowler NH, Dickinson M, Dreyling M, et al. Efficacy and safety of tisagenlecleucel in adult patients with relapsed/refractory follicular lymphoma: interim analysis of the phase 2 Elara Trial ASH Congress; 2020, abstract 1149.

Freeman CL, Kridel R, Moccia AA, et al. Early progression after bendamustine-rituximab is associated with high risk of transformation in advanced stage follicular lymphoma. Blood. 2019;134(9):761–4. https://doi.org/10.1182/blood.2019000258. Epub 2019 Jul 12.

Gopal AK, Kahl BS, Flowers CR, et al. Idelalisib is effective in patients with high-risk follicular lymphoma and early relapse after initial chemoimmunotherapy. Blood. 2017;129(22):3037–9. https://doi.org/10.1182/blood-2016-12-757740. Epub 2017 Mar 21.

Hutchings M, Mous R, Roost Clausen M, et al. Subcutaneous Epcoritamab induces complete responses with an encouraging safety profile across relapsed/refractory B-cell non-Hodgkin lymphoma subtypes, including patients with prior CAR-T therapy: updated dose escalation data. ASH Congress 2020a, abstract 402.

Hutchings M, Carlo-Stella C, Bachy E, et al. Glofitamab step-up dosing induces high response rates in patients with hard-to-treat refractory or relapsed non-Hodgkin lymphoma. ASH Congress; 2020b, abstract 403.

Jacobson C, Chavez JC, Sehgal AR, et al. Primary analysis of Zuma-5: a phase 2 study of Axicabtagene Ciloleucel (Axi-Cel) in patients with relapsed/refractory (R/R) indolent non-Hodgkin lymphoma (iNHL). ASH Congress; 2020, abstract700.

Kahl BS, Yang DT. Follicular lymphoma: evolving therapeutic strategies. Blood. 2016;127(17):2055–63. https://doi.org/10.1182/blood-2015-11-624288.

Leonard JP, Trneny M, Izutsu K, et al. AUGMENT: a phase III study of Lenalidomide plus rituximab versus placebo plus rituximab in relapsed or refractory indolent lymphoma. J Clin Oncol. 2019;37(14):1188–99. https://doi.org/10.1200/JCO.19.00010. Epub 2019 Mar 21.

Locke FL, Ghobadi A, Jacobson CA, et al. Long-term safety and activity of axicabtagene ciloleucel in refractory large B-cell lymphoma (ZUMA-1): a single-arm, multicentre, phase 1-2 trial. Lancet Oncol. 2019;20(1):31–42. https://doi.org/10.1016/S1470-2045(18)30864-7. Epub 2018 Dec 2.

Morschhauser F, Le Gouill S, Feugier P, et al. Obinutuzumab combined with lenalidomide for relapsed or refractory follicular B-cell lymphoma (GALEN): a multicentre, single-arm, phase 2 study. Lancet Haematol. 2019;6(8):e429–37. https://doi.org/10.1016/S2352-3026(19)30089-4. Epub 2019 Jul 8.

Neelapu SS, Locke FL, Bartlett NL, et al. Axicabtagene Ciloleucel CAR-T cell therapy in refractory large B-cell lymphoma. N Engl J Med. 2017;377(26):2531–44. https://doi.org/10.1056/NEJMoa1707447. Epub 2017 Dec 10.

Rivas-Delgado A, Laura Magnano L, Moreno-Velázquez M, et al. Response duration and survival shorten after each relapse in patients with follicular lymphoma treated in the rituximab era. Br J Haematol. 2019;184(5):753–9. https://doi.org/10.1111/bjh.15708. Epub 2018 Dec 4.

Sesques P, Bourcier J, Golfier C, et al. Clinical characteristics and outcomes of relapsed follicular lymphoma after autologous stem cell transplantation in the rituximab era. Hematol Oncol. 2020;38(2):137–45. https://doi.org/10.1002/hon.2713. Epub 2020 Jan 30.

Multiple Myeloma

16

Ibrahim Yakoub-Agha ⓘ and Hermann Einsele ⓘ

To date, over 100 clinical trials investigating the use of CAR-T cells in MM have been registered at clinicaltrials.gov. Although several CD19-directed CAR-T cell products have been approved (Ghobadi 2018; Yassine et al. 2020), CD19 surface expression on plasma cells is limited or absent, leading to uncertain efficacy in clinical trials that used anti-CD19 alone in patients with MM (Garfall et al. 2015, 2019). Using superresolution microscopy, CD19 can be detected on a large proportion of myeloma cells, which could explain the successful targeting and lysis of myeloma cells by CD19-detecting CAR-T cells (Nerreter et al. 2019). Of note, some ongoing studies in which CD19 is targeted in combination with other antigens, especially BCMA, are being conducted (Beauvais et al. 2020).

BCMA-directed CAR-T cells have shown promising efficacy and safety profiles in various phase I/II clinical trials (Munshi et al. 2021; Brudno et al. 2018; Cohen et al. 2019; Mailankody et al. 2020; Zhao et al. 2018). Indeed, the overall response rate ranged from 75 to 100%, with median event-free survival ranging from 11 to 24 months, in heavily pretreated MM patients, which is far better than all other currently available drugs and agents in this patient cohort.

At least two BCMA-directed CAR-T cell products will likely move into routine clinical use in the near future. Outside clinical trials, the main indication for CAR-T cell therapy in MM would be limited to patients with R/R MM after at least two lines of prior therapy that included PIs (proteasome inhibitors), iMIDs

I. Yakoub-Agha
Maladies du Sang, Unité de Thérapie Cellulaire, Centre hospitalier-Universitaire de Lille, Lille, France
e-mail: brahim.yakoubagha@chru-lille.fr

H. Einsele (✉)
Department of Internal Medicine II, University Hospital Würzburg, Würzburg, Bayern, Germany
e-mail: Einsele_H@ukw.de

(immunomodulatory agents, e.g., lenalidomide, pomalidomide), and anti-C38 monoclonal antibodies.

Although CAR-T cell therapy appears promising, the duration of disease control is limited, and almost all patients ultimately relapse. This might partially reflect the fact that CAR-T cells have thus far only been given to heavily pretreated patients with advanced, resistant disease (Beauvais et al. 2020; Gauthier and Yakoub-Agha 2017). Thus, CAR-T cell exhaustion and the reduction and even irreversible loss of expression of the target antigen BCMA on tumour cells (Da Vià et al. 2021; Samur et al. 2021), which are often genetically highly unstable, are other factors limiting CAR-T cell efficacy. Thus, novel targets or even dual targeting (including targeting of GPRC5D (de Larrea et al. 2020), SLAMF7 (Gogishvili et al. 2017), CD229 (Radhakrishnan et al. 2020), and CD38 (Gauthier and Yakoub-Agha 2017; Verkleij et al. 2020)) is currently being explored.

Additionally, to increase efficacy, CAR-T cell therapy is moved to earlier lines of therapy to increase the fitness and persistence of the generated MM-specific CAR-T cells. However, CAR-T cell therapy in MM—less when compared to patients with aggressive lymphomas—can be associated with substantial, potentially life-threatening toxicity. Thus, administering CAR-T cells with a better effector function and proliferation potential may be a challenge as CAR-T therapy is used at earlier stages of disease (Prommersberger et al. 2018).

> **Key Points**
> - BCMA is the major target for CAR-T cell therapy in MM.
> - Two BCMA-directed CAR-T cell products are moving into the clinical routine in the near future (one has already been approved by the FDA and EMA).
> - Irreversible BCMA loss on MM cells has been described in a few patients as a cause of failure of BCMA-directed CAR-T cells.
> - CAR-T cell therapy is moving to earlier lines of therapy in MM patients.

References

Beauvais D, Danhof S, Hayden PJ, Einsele H, Yakoub-Agha I. Clinical data, limitations and perspectives on chimeric antigen receptor T-cell therapy in multiple myeloma. Curr Opin Oncol. 2020;32(5):418–26.

Brudno JN, Maric I, Hartman SD, Rose JJ, Wang M, Lam N, Stetler-Stevenson M, Salem D, Yuan C, Pavletic S, et al. T cells genetically modified to express an anti-B-cell maturation antigen chimeric antigen receptor cause remissions of poor-prognosis relapsed multiple myeloma. J Clin Oncol. 2018;36(22):2267–80.

Cohen AD, Garfall AL, Stadtmauer EA, Melenhorst JJ, Lacey SF, Lancaster E, Vogl DT, Weiss BM, Dengel K, Nelson A, et al. B cell maturation antigen-specific CAR-T cells are clinically active in multiple myeloma. J Clin Invest. 2019;129(6):2210–21.

Da Vià MC, Dietrich O, Truger M, Arampatzi P, Duell J, Heidemeier A, Zhou X, Danhof S, Kraus S, Chatterjee M, Meggendorfer M, Twardziok S, Goebeler ME, Topp MS, Hudecek M, Prommersberger S, Hege K, Kaiser S, Fuhr V, Weinhold N, Rosenwald A, Erhard F, Haferlach C, Einsele H, Kortüm KM, Saliba AE, Rasche L. Homozygous BCMA gene deletion in response to anti-BCMA CAR-T cells in a patient with multiple myeloma. Nat Med. 2021;27(4):616–19.

Garfall AL, Maus MV, Hwang WT, Lacey SF, Mahnke YD, Melenhorst JJ, Zheng Z, Vogl DT, Cohen AD, Weiss BM, et al. Chimeric antigen receptor T cells against CD19 for multiple myeloma. N Engl J Med. 2015;373(11):1040–7.

Garfall AL, Stadtmauer EA, Hwang WT, Lacey SF, Melenhorst JJ, Krevvata M, Carroll MP, Matsui WH, Wang Q, Dhodapkar MV et al. Anti-CD19 CAR-T cells with high-dose melphalan and autologous stem cell transplantation for refractory multiple myeloma. JCI Insight. 2019;4(4):e127684.

Gauthier J, Yakoub-Agha I. Chimeric antigen-receptor T-cell therapy for hematological malignancies and solid tumors: clinical data to date, current limitations and perspectives. Curr Res Transl Med. 2017;65(3):93–102.

Ghobadi A. Chimeric antigen receptor T cell therapy for non-Hodgkin lymphoma. Curr Res Transl Med. 2018;66(2):43–9.

Gogishvili T, Danhof S, Prommersberger S, Rydzek J, Schreder M, Brede C, Einsele H, Hudecek M. SLAMF7-CAR-T cells eliminate myeloma and confer selective fratricide of SLAMF7(+) normal lymphocytes. Blood. 2017;130(26):2838–47.

de Larrea CF, Staehr M, Lopez AV, Ng KY, Chen Y, Godfrey WD, Purdon TJ, Ponomarev V, Wendel HG, Brentjens RJ, Smith EL. Defining an optimal dual-targeted CAR-T cell therapy approach simultaneously targeting BCMA and GPRC5D to prevent BCMA escape-driven relapse in multiple myeloma. Blood Cancer Discov. 2020;1(2):146–54.

Mailankody S, Jakubowiak AJ, Htut M, Costa LJ, Lee K, Ganguly S, Kaufman JL, Siegel DSD, Bensinger W, Cota M, et al. Orvacabtagene autoleucel (orva-cel), a B-cell maturation antigen (BCMA)-directed CAR-T cell therapy for patients (pts) with relapsed/refractory multiple myeloma (RRMM): update of the phase 1/2 EVOLVE study (NCT03430011). J Clin Oncol. 2020;38(15_Suppl):8504.

Munshi NC, Anderson LD Jr, Shah N, Madduri D, Berdeja J, Lonial S, Raje N, Lin Y, Siegel D, Oriol A, et al. Idecabtagene Vicleucel in relapsed and refractory multiple myeloma. N Engl J Med. 2021;384(8):705–16.

Nerreter T, Letschert S, Götz R, Doose S, Danhof S, Einsele H, Sauer M, Hudecek M. Super-resolution microscopy reveals ultra-low CD19 expression on myeloma cells that triggers elimination by CD19 CAR-T. Nat Commun. 2019;10(1):3137.

Prommersberger S, Jetani H, Danhof S, Monjezi R, Nerreter T, Beckmann J, Einsele H, Hudecek M. Novel targets and technologies for CAR-T cells in multiple myeloma and acute myeloid leukemia. Curr Res Transl Med. 2018;66(2):37–8.

Radhakrishnan SV, Luetkens T, Scherer SD, Davis P, Vander Mause ER, Olson ML, Yousef S, Panse J, Abdiche Y, Li KD, Miles RR, Matsui W, Welm AL, Atanackovic D. CD229 CAR-T cells eliminate multiple myeloma and tumor propagating cells without fratricide. Nat Commun. 2020;11(1):798.

Samur MK, Fulciniti M, Aktas Samur A, Bazarbachi AH, Tai YT, Prabhala R, Alonso A, Sperling AS, Campbell T, Petrocca F, Hege K, Kaiser S, Loiseau HA, Anderson KC, Munshi NC. Biallelic loss of BCMA as a resistance mechanism to CAR-T cell therapy in a patient with multiple myeloma. Nat Commun. 2021;12(1):868.

Verkleij CPM, Jhatakia A, Broekmans MEC, Frerichs KA, Zweegman S, Mutis T, Bezman NA, van de Donk NWCJ. Preclinical rationale for targeting the PD-1/PD-L1 Axis in combination with a CD38 antibody in multiple myeloma and other CD38-positive malignancies. Cancers (Basel). 2020;12(12):3713.

Yassine F, Iqbal M, Murthy H, Kharfan-Dabaja MA, Chavez JC. Real world experience of approved chimeric antigen receptor T-cell therapies outside of clinical trials. Curr Res Transl Med. 2020;68(4):159–70.

Zhao WH, Liu J, Wang BY, Chen YX, Cao XM, Yang Y, Zhang YL, Wang FX, Zhang PY, Lei B, et al. A phase 1, open-label study of LCAR-B38M, a chimeric antigen receptor T cell therapy directed against B cell maturation antigen, in patients with relapsed or refractory multiple myeloma. J Hematol Oncol. 2018;11(1):141.

Developments in Other Haematological Malignancies: Other Lymphoid Malignancies

Paolo Corradini and Lorenz Trümper

Peripheral T cell lymphomas comprise a heterogeneous group of rare diseases, representing 10–15% of all non-Hodgkin lymphomas (NHLs). Upfront treatment for peripheral T cell lymphoma (pTNHL) includes CHOP-like (cyclophosphamide, adriamycin, vincristine, prednisone) multiagent chemotherapy with or without etoposide, followed by stem cell transplantation as consolidation in responsive fit patients. This approach induces durable long-term remission in approximately 40% of cases; early refractoriness during induction occurs in approximately 25% of patients, with the remaining patients typically relapsing within 24 months. With the exception of patients with anaplastic large cell lymphomas who are eligible to receive brentuximab vedotin, there is no standard of care in the relapse setting. In patients not eligible to receive high-dose chemotherapy followed by allogeneic stem cell transplantation, the prognosis is dismal.

CAR-T cells have shown impressive results in relapsed/refractory B-cell lymphoma and are currently under investigation in T cell lymphomas.

Target Antigens

The choice of the appropriate antigen constitutes the main challenge in targeting T cell malignancies using CAR-T cells. Many target antigens are expressed by both physiological T cells and engineered CAR-T cells (Tables 17.1 and 17.2).

P. Corradini
Divisione di Ematologia, Fondazione IRCCS Istituto Nazionale dei Tumori di Milano, Università degli Studi di Milano, Milan, Italy
e-mail: paolo.corradini@unimi.it

L. Trümper (✉)
Department of Hematology and Oncology, Georg-August University Göttingen, Göttingen, Germany
e-mail: lorenz.truemper@med.uni-goettingen.de

© The Author(s) 2022
N. Kröger et al. (eds.), *The EBMT/EHA CAR-T Cell Handbook*,
https://doi.org/10.1007/978-3-030-94353-0_17

91

Table 17.1 Pan-T cell antigens

CD5	Expression in T cells, thymocytes, B-1 cells, and T cell malignancies:
	90% T-ALL/Ly
	85% PTCL-nos
	96% AITL
	26–32% ALCL
	36% NK-T
	85% ATLL
	91% CTCL
CD7	Expression in T cells, thymocytes, NK cells, and T cell malignancies:
	95% T-ALL/Ly
	50% PTCL-nos
	57% AITL
	32–54% ALCL
	79% NK-T
	25% ATLL
	18% CTCL

Table 17.2 Antigens with restricted expression

CD30	Expression in activated T and B cells and in T cell malignancies:
	17% T-ALL/Ly
	16% PTCL-nos
	32–50% AITL
	93% ALCL
	64% NK-T
	39% ATLL
	18% CTCL
TRBC1	Expression in T cells and in T cell malignancies:
	7–11% T-ALL/Ly
	27% PTCL-nos
	34% AITL
	25% ALCL

Therefore, this shared antigen expression can potentially result in the following issues:

- A fratricide effect on CAR-T cells.
- Ablation of physiological donor T cells after CAR-T cell infusion, leading to deep and/or long-lasting immune deficiency and T cell aplasia.

CAR-T Development in T Cell Malignancies

Some experimentally engineered CAR-T cell products targeting CD5, CD7, CD30, and TRBC1 (T cell receptor beta chain 1) have been tested (Table 17.3).

Table 17.3 CAR-T cells targeting T lymphocyte antigens

CAR-T cells targeting CD5	*Mamonkin* et al. (Blood 2015), preclinical experience: – CD5 CAR-T cells eliminate malignant T-ALL/Ly lines in vitro and inhibit disease progression in xenograft mouse models – Second-generation CD5 CAR with a CD28 costimulatory domain: With the loss of CD5 expression on the surface of T cells, CD5 CAR-T cells become resistant to fratricide *Hill* et al. (Blood 2019), phase I dose escalation study, MAGENTA trial: – 9 patients enrolled (4 T-ALL, 5 T-NHL) – CD5 CAR-T cells are safe and can induce clinical responses (3 patients in complete response) in heavily pretreated relapsed/refractory T-ALL and T-NHL, without inducing T cell aplasia
CAR-T cells targeting CD7	*Gomes-Silva* et al. (Blood 2017), preclinical models of T cell malignancies: – Fulminant fratricide precluding expansion of CAR-T cells – Abrogation of CD7 expression from the cell surface shows potential activity A phase I study (CRIMSON trial) has been designed at Baylor College of Medicine but is not yet recruiting
CAR-T cells targeting TRBC1	*Maciocia* et al. (Nat Med 2017), preclinical studies: – CAR-T cells targeting TRBC1 are able to specifically eliminate malignant T cell lines expressing TRBC1 – TRBC1 CAR-T cells cannot target normal TRBC2-positive T cells A phase I/II study (AUTO4) coordinated by the University College of London is a single-arm trial evaluating the safety and clinical activity of a CAR-T cell targeting TRBC1 in patients with relapsed/refractory TRBC1-positive T cell lymphomas
CAR-T cells targeting CD30	*Dotti* et al. (Immunol Rev. 2014), preclinical studies: – CAR-T cells targeting CD30 generate tumour-specific T cells in patients with Hodgkin and anaplastic T cell lymphomas – Tumour recognition by CD30 CAR-T cells is MHC-unrestricted – CAR-T cells targeting CD30 potentially overcome tumour escape Several small clinical trials are being reported; some studies are ongoing and recruiting: – Two CAR-T constructs are under investigation, one CAR-T cell with the antigen-binding domain of the anti-CD30 and ant-CD28 costimulatory domain and another CAR-T cell targeting CD30 and 4-1BB as a costimulatory domain – In the *Ramos* et al. phase I study, 9 patients with relapsed/refractory Hodgkin and EBV-negative, CD30-positive ALCL have been treated; results are promising, with 1 patient in complete remission and 3 in stable disease, without relevant toxicities – *Wang* et al. enrolled 18 patients (17 Hodgkin, one ALCL); seven patients achieved a partial response and six achieved stable disease, with limited acute toxicities but an increased risk of infections – *Grover* et al. enrolled 24 patients (Hodgkin, ALCL, EATL, and Sezary syndrome) in a phase Ib/II study with anti-CD30 CAR-T cells, which demonstrated early clinical effects and good tolerability and safety – A phase I study is ongoing at the National Cancer Institute to assess safety and feasibility in advanced CD30-positive ALCL and PTCL-NOS

Key Points
- Target antigens are expressed by normal T cells, malignant T cells, and engineered CAR-T cells.
- Therefore, the major concern for targeting T cell malignancies with CAR-T cells is a fratricide effect.
- A second major issue is the ablation of normal T cells after CAR-T cell infusion, potentially causing severe and/or long-lasting immune deficiency and T cell aplasia.
- Currently, the most promising constructs are CAR-T cells targeting CD30.
- Phase I and II studies are ongoing in T cell malignancies and Hodgkin lymphoma, thus far demonstrating feasibility, tolerability, and potential for clinical efficacy.

Bibliography

Dotti G, Gottschalk S, Savoldo B, et al. Design and development of therapies using chimeric antigen receptor-expressing T cells. Immunol Rev. 2014;257(1):107–26.

Foster C, Kuruvilla J. Treatment approaches in relapsed or refractory peripheral T-cell lymphomas. F1000Research. 2020;9(Faculty Rev):1091.

Gomes-Silva D, Srinivasan M, Sharma S, et al. CD7-edited T cells expressing a CD7-specific CAR for the therapy of T-cell malignancies. Blood. 2017;130:285–96.

Grover NS, Park SI, Ivanova A, et al. A phase Ib/II study of anti-CD30 chimeric antigen receptor T cells for relapsed/refractory CD30+ lymphomas. Biol Blood Marrow Transplant. 2019;25(3):S66.

Hill LC, Rouce RH, Smith TS, et al. Safety and anti-tumor activity of CD5 CAR-T cells in patients with relapsed/refractory T-cell malignancies. Blood. 2019;134(S1):199.

Maciocia PM, Wawrzyniecka PA, Philip B, et al. Targeting the T cell receptor β-chain constant region for immunotherapy of T cell malignancies. Nat Med. 2017;23(12):1416–23.

Mamonkin M, Rouce RH, Tashiro H, et al. A T-cell directed chimeric antigen receptor for the selective treatment of T-cell malignancies. Blood. 2015;126:983–92.

Ramos CA, Ballard B, Zhang H, et al. Clinical and immunological responses after CD30-specific chimeric antigen receptor–redirected lymphocytes. J Clin Invest. 2017;127(9):3462–71.

Rogers AM, Brammer JE. Hematopoietic cell transplantation and adoptive cell therapy in peripheral T cell lymphoma. Curr Hematol Malig Rep. 2020;15:316–32.

Sherer LD, Brenner MK, Mamonkin M. Chimeric antigen receptors for T-cell malignancies. Front Oncol. 2019;9(126):1–10.

Vose J, Armitage J, Weisenburger D. International peripheral T-cell and natural killer/T-cell lymphoma study: pathology findings and clinical outcomes. J Clin Oncol. 2008;26(25):4124–30.

Wang CM, Wu ZQ, Wang Y, et al. Autologous T cells expressing CD30 chimeric antigen receptors for relapsed or refractory Hodgkin lymphoma: an open-label phase I trial. Clin Cancer Res. 2017;23(5):1156–66.

Myeloid Malignancies

18

Christophe Ferrand and Alessandro Rambaldi

In addition to chemotherapy, which remains the basic treatment, the treatment panel for acute myeloid leukaemia (AML) has expanded considerably in recent years. Clinicians now have a large choice of therapies: targeted therapies (anti-IDH1/2, anti-FLT3, and anti-BCL2 therapies, among others), drugs targeting epigenetic mechanisms, kinase inhibitors (FLT3, MAPK, and JAK2, etc.), immunotherapies (monoclonal antibodies linked or not to a toxin, dual/bispecific), and cellular immunotherapies. Moreover, despite its toxicities, allogeneic transplantation often remains an effective final therapeutic alternative. However, most patients are refractory or relapsed (R/R) after several lines of therapy. Thus, there is a clinical need in AML R/R patients, and CAR-T cells may be an option and can find a place in the treatment to reduce tumour burden and clinical evolution of the disease (Fig. 18.1, modified from Roussel et al. (2020)).

Several currently ongoing research programs aim to generate CAR-T cells against myeloid malignancies (Hofmann et al. 2019). However, the absence of a truly AML-specific marker generates remarkable uncertainty regarding the optimal antigens to target, and significant concern remains about off-target effects on normal haematopoiesis. The difficulty of obtaining successful manufacture of CAR-T cells from heavily pretreated patients has paved the way to investigation of different cell sources to build alternative platforms for cellular therapy.

C. Ferrand
EFS – INSERM UMR1098 RIGHT – UBFC, Molecular Onco Hematology Lab, EFS Bourgogne Franche-Comté, Besançon, France
e-mail: christophe.ferrand@efs.sante.fr

A. Rambaldi (✉)
Department of Oncology-Hematology, University of Milan and Azienda Socio Sanitaria Territoriale Papa Giovanni XXIII, Bergamo, Italy
e-mail: alessandro.rambaldi@unimi.it

© The Author(s) 2022
N. Kröger et al. (eds.), *The EBMT/EHA CAR-T Cell Handbook*,
https://doi.org/10.1007/978-3-030-94353-0_18

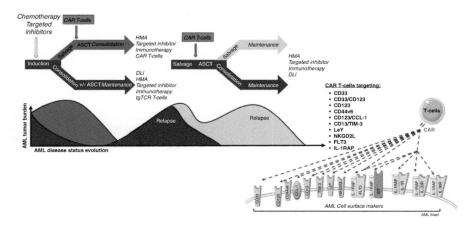

Fig. 18.1 Putative place of CAR-T cells in the AML treatment strategy. *HMA* hypomethylated agent, *DLI* donor lymphocyte infusion, *tgTCR* transgenic T cell receptor T cells, *ASCT* allogeneic stem cell transplantation

Single or Dual Antigen Targeting?

CAR-T cells targeting CD33 and CD123 have already been investigated in early phase clinical trials. Unfortunately, these antigens do not avoid "on-target off-tumour" effects, such as myelotoxicity and endothelial toxicity. For this reason, CAR-T cells directed against other surface proteins, such as CCL-1, CD44v6, FLT3, c-KIT (CD117), CD38, B7-H3 (also known as CD276), NKG2D, and IL-1RAP, are also under preclinical and clinical investigation (Table 18.1).

CD123 CAR-T cells induce haematopoietic toxicity but on a smaller scale than CD33 CAR-T cells, particularly following anti-CD123 single chain fragment variable (scFv) modifications (Mardiros et al. 2013; Gill et al. 2014; Thokala et al. 2016). Nevertheless, based on their expression on stem cells, CD123 CAR-T cells could be used as a myeloablative regimen before ASCT, thus representing an interesting strategy for treatment of R/R AML patients (Gill et al. 2014; Cummins and Gill 2019; Testa et al. 2019). Notably, IL-15 may enhance the anti-AML activity of CD123 CAR-T cells (Mu-Mosley et al. 2019). Targeting FLT3 or CD117 could be an attractive option, again in association with ASCT (Jetani et al. 2018; Myburgh et al. 2020). Targeting of the Lewis Y antigen and NKG2DL CAR-T cells has also been proposed, but phase 1 trials have shown short response durations, despite reduced toxicity (Ritchie et al. 2013; Driouk et al. 2019). CAR-T cells targeting CD44v6 mediate potent antitumour effects against AML while sparing normal haematopoietic stem cells (Casucci et al. 2013), and a clinical trial is currently ongoing. A potent effect on LSCs was observed with CAR-T cells targeting IL1RAP (Warda et al. 2019) with no apparent effect on healthy haematopoietic stem cells. Similar more specific antileukaemic activity was observed by targeting FLT3 and KIT mutations (Mitchell et al. 2018). Interestingly, targeting IL1RAP decreases IL-1, IL-6, IL-10, IL-13, IL-17, IL-22, IFNγ, and TNFα levels (Højen et al. 2019). The

Table 18.1 CAR-T cell immunotherapies under investigation in AML (based on www.clinicaltrials.gov at 05/25/2020)

CAR-T cells	Preclinical results	Status	Clinical trials
CD33	Myeloablative, ASCT requirement	Phase 1	NCT03126864
		Phase 1/2	NCT03971799, NCT01864902
CD123	Myeloablative, ASCT requirement	Phase 1	NCT03796390, NCT03585517, NCT03114670, NCT03766126, NCT04014881, NCT03190278, NCT02159495, NCT04230265, NCT04318678, NCT03672851
		Phase 1/2	NCT04272125, NCT04265963, NCT04109482, NCT03556982
CCL-1	AML and HSC targeting	Phase 1	NCT04219163
CD38	AML targeting	Phase 1/2	NCT04351022
CD44v6	AML targeting	Phase 1/2	NCT04097301
FLT3	Myeloablative, ASCT requirement	Phase 1	NCT03904069
KIT (CD117)	Myeloablative, ASCT requirement	Preclinical	NCT03473457
B7-H3	HSC toxicity reduction	Preclinical	None
CD13 TIM-3	HSC toxicity reduction	Preclinical	None
PD-1	Antitumour enhancement	Preclinical	None
Lewis Y	Short duration of response, few toxicities	Phase 1	*NCT01716364, no further study*
NKGD2L	Short duration of response, few toxicities	Phase 1	*NCT02203825, no further study*
IL1RAP	LSC targeting	Preclinical	NCT04169022
CD33/CD123	AML and HSC targeting	Phase 1	NCT04156256
CCL-1/CD123	AML targeting	Phase 2/3	NCT03631576
CCL-1/CD33	AML targeting	Phase 1	NCT03795779
CCL-1/CD33 and/or CD123	AML targeting	Phase 1/2	NCT04010877
Muc1/CLL1/ CD33/CD38/ CD56/ CD123	AML targeting	Phase 1/2	NCT03222674

Studies investigating T cell immunotherapies in AML. *AML* acute myeloid leukaemia, *LSC* leukaemic stem cell, *HSC* haematopoietic stem cell, *ASCT* allogeneic stem cell transplantation

reduced production of IL-4, IL-6 and IL-10 and absence of IL-17 production (Warda et al. 2019) may in turn limit CAR-T cell cytokine release syndrome (CRS) and the immune effector cell-associated neurotoxicity syndrome (ICAN) associated with excessive production of IL-1 (Garcia Borrega et al. 2019). Notably, the reduction in IL-1β, IL-6, and TNFα levels leads to decreased release of IL-10 and TGFβ, which impair CAR-T cell functions (Epperly et al. 2020).

CAR-T cells simultaneously targeting CD33 and CD123 are also in development and exhibit pronounced antileukaemic activity (Petrov et al. 2018). Similarly, CD123 and CCL-1 compound CAR-T cells may be useful for active targeting of leukaemia stem cells (LSCs) (Morsink et al. 2018; Shang and Zhou 2019).

Bispecific CD13-TIM-3 CAR-T cells (He et al. 2020) and B7-H3 CAR-T cells (Lichtman et al. 2018) showed reduced HSC toxicity. Moreover, the B7-H3 pan-cancer target was also studied in solid tumours (Waldman et al. 2020). Preliminary reports show that PD-1 inhibitors also regulate the CAR-T cell response, although few data are available. Furthermore, delivery of PD-1-blocking scFv CAR-T cells in preclinical investigations demonstrated interesting antitumour efficacy enhancement (Anonymous 2019). Several challenges remain to be overcome, as recently reported, and further investigations may provide a better understanding (Mardiana and Gill 2020).

Molecular Engineering of the Chimeric Receptor and Alternative Cell Sources

Beyond the selected target, optimizing the molecular engineering of the chimeric receptor remains crucial. CD33 4-1BBz CAR-T cells have shown antileukaemic activity and resistance to exhaustion with increasing central memory comportment (Li et al. 2018). An additional strategy that has been proposed to reduce haematopoietic toxicity is the use of a transiently expressed CART33 to induce self-limiting activity against AML cells (Kenderian et al. 2015). Another proposed strategy is to inactivate the *CD33* gene in HSCs prior to transplantation to prevent CD33-induced haematopoietic toxicity of CAR-T cells (Kim et al. 2018).

In addition, to avoid or reduce the uncontrolled toxicity of expanding CAR-T cells, the use of the anti-CD52 antibody alemtuzumab or a suicide gene strategy based on CD20 protein coexpression in CD123 CAR-T cells has been proposed for subsequent anti-CD20 targeting with rituximab (Introna et al. 2000; Tasian et al. 2017).

Several clinical trials are currently evaluating the use of allogeneic CAR-T cells in haematologic malignancies, employing different effector cell types, such as NK cells (Daher and Rezvani 2021) or TCR-edited cells (Provasi et al. 2012), to limit GvHD and develop strategies to avoid the rejection of allogeneic cells. In this regard, the limited GvHD associated with the use of cytokine-induced killer (CIK) cells (Martino Introna et al. 2017) was confirmed in a phase I/IIa study in which B-ALL patients who relapsed after allogeneic transplantation were treated using CD19-specific CAR CIK cells (CARCIK-CD19) manufactured from a previous transplant donor (Magnani et al. 2020). Notably, this study provides evidence of the feasibility of employing a nonviral sleeping beauty transposon system to successfully produce CARCIK cell products starting from a small amount of donor-derived PB, thus offering a valid alternative to viral vectors. The use of CAR-engineered CIK cells was also demonstrated to be effective for AML by characterizing the targeting of the two most validated AML molecules, CD33 and CD123, in vitro and in vivo (Tettamanti et al. 2013; Pizzitola et al. 2014; Arcangeli et al. 2017; Rotiroti et al. 2020).

> **Key Points**
> - The primary challenge limiting the use of CAR-T cells in myeloid malignancies is the absence of an ideal antigen.
> - Myeloid antigens are often coexpressed on normal haematopoietic stem/progenitor cells (HSPCs).
> - Myelotoxicity and endothelial toxicity can be overcome by "and/or" dual CAR targeting.
> - Allogeneic CAR-T cells may be a future alternative.

References

Anonymous. Augmenting CAR-T cells with PD-1 blockade. Cancer Discov. 2019;9(2): 158. https://doi.org/10.1158/2159-8290.CD-NB2018-165.

Arcangeli S, Rotiroti MC, Bardelli M, Simonelli L, Magnani CF, Biondi A, Biagi E, Tettamanti S, Varani L. Balance of anti-CD123 chimeric antigen receptor binding affinity and density for the targeting of acute myeloid leukemia. Mol Ther. 2017;25(8):1933–45. https://doi.org/10.1016/j.ymthe.2017.04.017.

Borrega G, Jorge PG, Rüger MA, Onur ÖA, Shimabukuro-Vornhagen A, Kochanek M, Böll B. In the eye of the storm: immune-mediated toxicities associated with CAR-T cell therapy. HemaSphere. 2019;3(2):e191. https://doi.org/10.1097/HS9.0000000000000191.

Casucci M, di Robilant BN, Falcone L, Camisa B, Norelli M, Genovese P, Gentner B, et al. CD44v6-targeted T cells mediate potent antitumor effects against acute myeloid leukemia and multiple myeloma. Blood. 2013;122(20):3461–72. https://doi.org/10.1182/blood-2013-04-493361.

Cummins KD, Gill S. Chimeric antigen receptor T-cell therapy for acute myeloid leukemia: how close to reality? Haematologica. 2019;104(7):1302–8. https://doi.org/10.3324/haematol.2018.208751.

Daher M, Rezvani K. Outlook for new CAR-based therapies with a focus on CAR NK cells: what lies beyond CAR-engineered T cells in the race against cancer. Cancer Discov. 2021;11(1):45–58. https://doi.org/10.1158/2159-8290.CD-20-0556.

Driouk L, Gicobi J, Kamihara Y, Rutherford K, Dranoff G, Ritz J, Baumeister SHC. Chimeric antigen receptor T cells targeting NKG2D-ligands show robust efficacy against acute myeloid leukemia and T-cell acute lymphoblastic leukemia. Blood. 2019;134(Suppl 1):1930. https://doi.org/10.1182/blood-2019-130113.

Epperly R, Gottschalk S, Paulina Velasquez M. A bump in the road: how the hostile AML microenvironment affects CAR-T cell therapy. Front Oncol. 2020;10:262. https://doi.org/10.3389/fonc.2020.00262.

Gill S, Tasian SK, Ruella M, Shestova O, Li Y, Porter DL, Carroll M, et al. Preclinical targeting of human acute myeloid leukemia and myeloablation using chimeric antigen receptor-modified T cells. Blood. 2014;123(15):2343–54. https://doi.org/10.1182/blood-2013-09-529537.

He X, Feng Z, Ma J, Ling S, Cao Y, Gurung B, Wu Y, et al. Bispecific and split CAR-T cells targeting CD13 and TIM3 eradicate acute myeloid leukemia. Blood. 2020;135(10):713–23. https://doi.org/10.1182/blood.2019002779.

Hofmann S, Schubert M-L, Wang L, He B, Neuber B, Dreger P, Müller-Tidow C, Schmitt M. Chimeric antigen receptor (CAR) T cell therapy in acute myeloid leukemia (AML). J Clin Med. 2019;8(2):200. https://doi.org/10.3390/jcm8020200.

Højen JF, Kristensen MLV, McKee AS, Wade MT, Azam T, Lunding LP, de Graaf DM, et al. IL-1R3 blockade broadly attenuates the functions of six members of the IL-1 family, revealing their contribution to models of disease. Nat Immunol. 2019;20(9):1138–49. https://doi.org/10.1038/s41590-019-0467-1.

Introna M, Barbui AM, Bambacioni F, Casati C, Gaipa G, Borleri G, Bernasconi S, et al. Genetic modification of human T cells with CD20: a strategy to purify and lyse transduced cells with anti-CD20 antibodies. Hum Gene Ther. 2000;11(4):611–20. https://doi.org/10.1089/10430340050015798.

Introna M, Lussana F, Algarotti A, Gotti E, Valgardsdottir R, Mico C, Grassi A, et al. Phase II study of sequential infusion of donor lymphocyte infusion and cytokine-induced killer cells for patients relapsed after allogeneic hematopoietic stem cell transplantation. Biol Blood Marrow Transplant. 2017;23(12):2070–8. https://doi.org/10.1016/j.bbmt.2017.07.005.

Jetani H, Garcia-Cadenas I, Nerreter T, Thomas S, Rydzek J, Meijide JB, Bonig H, et al. CAR-T cells targeting FLT3 have potent activity against FLT3(−)ITD(+) AML and act synergistically with the FLT3-inhibitor crenolanib. Leukemia. 2018;32(5):1168–79. https://doi.org/10.1038/s41375-018-0009-0.

Kenderian SS, Ruella M, Shestova O, Klichinsky M, Aikawa V, Morrissette JJD, Scholler J, et al. CD33-specific chimeric antigen receptor T cells exhibit potent preclinical activity against human acute myeloid leukemia. Leukemia. 2015;29(8):1637–47. https://doi.org/10.1038/leu.2015.52.

Kim MY, Kyung-Rok Y, Kenderian SS, Ruella M, Chen S, Shin T-H, Aljanahi AA, et al. Genetic inactivation of CD33 in hematopoietic stem cells to enable CAR-T cell immunotherapy for acute myeloid leukemia. Cell. 2018;173(6):1439–1453.e19. https://doi.org/10.1016/j.cell.2018.05.013.

Li S, Tao Z, Yingxi X, Liu J, An N, Wang Y, Xing H, et al. CD33-specific chimeric antigen receptor T cells with different co-stimulators showed potent anti-leukemia efficacy and different phenotype. Hum Gene Ther. 2018;29(5):626–39. https://doi.org/10.1089/hum.2017.241.

Lichtman E, Hongwei D, Savoldo B, Ferrone S, Li G, Lishan S, Dotti G. Pre-clinical evaluation of B7-H3-specific chimeric antigen receptor T-cells for the treatment of acute myeloid leukemia. Blood. 2018;132(Suppl 1):701. https://doi.org/10.1182/blood-2018-99-113468.

Magnani CF, Gaipa G, Lussana F, Belotti D, Gritti G, Napolitano S, Matera G, et al. Sleeping beauty–engineered CAR-T cells achieve antileukemic activity without severe toxicities. J Clin Invest. 2020;130(11):6021–33. https://doi.org/10.1172/JCI138473.

Mardiana S, Gill S. CAR-T cells for acute myeloid leukemia: state of the art and future directions. Front Oncol. 2020;10:697. https://doi.org/10.3389/fonc.2020.00697.

Mardiros A, Dos Santos C, McDonald T, Brown CE, Xiuli Wang L, Budde E, Hoffman L, et al. T cells expressing CD123-specific chimeric antigen receptors exhibit specific cytolytic effector functions and antitumor effects against human acute myeloid leukemia. Blood. 2013;122(18):3138–48. https://doi.org/10.1182/blood-2012-12-474056.

Mitchell K, Barreyro L, Todorova TI, Taylor SJ, Antony-Debré I, Narayanagari S-R, Carvajal LA, et al. IL1RAP potentiates multiple oncogenic signaling pathways in AML. J Exp Med. 2018;215(6):1709–27. https://doi.org/10.1084/jem.20180147.

Morsink L, Walter R, Ossenkoppele G. Prognostic and therapeutic role of CLEC12A in acute myeloid leukemia. Blood Rev. 2018;34:26–33. https://doi.org/10.1016/j.blre.2018.10.003.

Mu-Mosley H, Ostermann LB, Muftuoglu M, Schober W, Patel NB, Vaidya A, Bonifant CL, Gottschalk S, Velasquez MP, Andreeff M. Transgenic expression of IL15 in CD123-specific BiTE-secreting engager T-cells results in improved anti-AML activity. Blood. 2019;134(Suppl 1):3917. https://doi.org/10.1182/blood-2019-125928.

Myburgh R, Kiefer JD, Russkamp NF, Magnani CF, Nuñez N, Simonis A, Pfister S, et al. Anti-human CD117 CAR-T cells efficiently eliminate healthy and malignant CD117-expressing hematopoietic cells. Leukemia. 2020;34(10):2688–703. https://doi.org/10.1038/s41375-020-0818-9.

Petrov JC, Wada M, Pinz KG, Yan LE, Chen KH, Shuai X, Liu H, et al. Compound CAR-T cells as a double-pronged approach for treating acute myeloid leukemia. Leukemia. 2018;32(6):1317–26. https://doi.org/10.1038/s41375-018-0075-3.

Pizzitola I, Anjos-Afonso F, Rouault-Pierre K, Lassailly F, Tettamanti S, Spinelli O, Biondi A, Biagi E, Bonnet D. Chimeric antigen receptors against CD33/CD123 antigens efficiently target primary acute myeloid leukemia cells in vivo. Leukemia. 2014;28(8):1596–605. https://doi. org/10.1038/leu.2014.62.

Provasi E, Genovese P, Lombardo A, Magnani Z, Liu P-Q, Reik A, Chu V, et al. Editing T cell specificity towards leukemia by zinc finger nucleases and lentiviral gene transfer. Nat Med. 2012;18(5):807–15. https://doi.org/10.1038/nm.2700.

Ritchie DS, Neeson PJ, Khot A, Peinert S, Tai T, Tainton K, Chen K, et al. Persistence and efficacy of second generation CAR-T cell against the LeY antigen in acute myeloid leukemia. Mol Ther. 2013;21(11):2122–9. https://doi.org/10.1038/mt.2013.154.

Rotiroti MC, Buracchi C, Arcangeli S, Galimberti S, Valsecchi MG, Perriello VM, Rasko T, et al. Targeting CD33 in chemoresistant AML patient-derived xenografts by CAR-CIK cells modified with an improved SB transposon system. Mol Ther. 2020;28(9):1974–86. https://doi. org/10.1016/j.ymthe.2020.05.021.

Roussel X, Daguindau E, Berceanu A, Desbrosses Y, Warda W, Neto M, da Rocha R, Trad ED, Deschamps M, Ferrand C. Acute myeloid leukemia: from biology to clinical practices through development and pre-clinical therapeutics. Front Oncol. 2020;10:599933. https://doi. org/10.3389/fonc.2020.599933.

Shang Y, Zhou F. Current advances in immunotherapy for acute leukemia: an overview of antibody, chimeric antigen receptor, immune checkpoint, and natural killer. Front Oncol. 2019;9:917. https:// doi.org/10.3389/fonc.2019.00917.

Tasian SK, Kenderian SS, Shen F, Ruella M, Shestova O, Kozlowski M, Li Y, et al. Optimized depletion of chimeric antigen receptor T cells in murine xenograft models of human acute myeloid leukemia. Blood. 2017;129(17):2395–407. https://doi.org/10.1182/blood-2016-08-736041.

Testa U, Pelosi E, Castelli G. CD123 as a therapeutic target in the treatment of hematological malignancies. Cancers. 2019;11(9):1358. https://doi.org/10.3390/cancers11091358.

Tettamanti S, Marin V, Pizzitola I, Magnani CF, Giordano GMP, Attianese EC, Maltese F, et al. Targeting of acute myeloid leukaemia by cytokine-induced killer cells redirected with a novel CD123-specific chimeric antigen receptor. Br J Haematol. 2013;161(3):389–401. https://doi. org/10.1111/bjh.12282.

Thokala R, Olivares S, Mi T, Maiti S, Deniger D, Huls H, Torikai H, et al. Redirecting specificity of T cells using the sleeping beauty system to express chimeric antigen receptors by mix-and-matching of VL and VH domains targeting CD123+ tumors. PLoS One. 2016;11(8):e0159477.

Waldman AD, Fritz JM, Lenardo MJ. A guide to cancer immunotherapy: from T cell basic science to clinical practice. Nat Rev Immunol. 2020;20(11):651–68. https://doi.org/10.1038/ s41577-020-0306-5.

Warda W, Larosa F, Da Rocha MN, Trad R, Deconinck E, Fajloun Z, Faure C, et al. CML hematopoietic stem cells expressing IL1RAP can be targeted by chimeric antigen receptor–engineered T cells. Cancer Res. 2019;79(3):663–75. https://doi.org/10.1158/0008-5472.CAN-18-1078.

Developments in Solid Tumours

19

Paolo Pedrazzoli and John B. A. G. Haanen

Chimeric antigen receptor (CAR) T cells have emerged as breakthrough therapies in patients with refractory haematologic malignancies, and the highly encouraging clinical results have fuelled expectations of implementing these strategies in other cancer types. However, a similar success of CAR-T cell treatment has not yet been observed in solid tumours. Various factors, including the immunosuppressive nature of the tumour microenvironment, hinder of CAR-T cell trafficking and infiltration into scarcely accessible tumour sites, and difficulties in identifying targetable antigens with optimal expression and a good toxicity profile, and limiting CAR-T dose escalation, must be overcome to achieve success in the treatment of solid cancers (Comoli et al. 2019).

Several clinical trials have tested the efficacy of CAR-T cells in solid tumours. To date, clinical results have not been encouraging, with a general lack of therapeutic response and the presence of on-target off-tumour toxicity. However, some studies have achieved promising outcomes that justify further exploration of this approach in solid tumours, as is happening in many areas of the world (Comoli et al. 2019).

Early experiences with GD2-specific CAR-T cells showed objective responses in paediatric patients with neuroblastoma (Pule et al. 2008). Since then, lymphocytes have been engineered via insertion of third-generation CARs and, more recently, by delivery of a GD2-CAR-IL-15 construct to NK cells (Heczey et al. 2020).

P. Pedrazzoli
Oncology Unit, Fondazione IRCCS Policlinico San Matteo, Department of Internal Medicine and Medical Therapy, University of Pavia, Pavia, Italy
e-mail: p.pedrazzoli@smatteo.pv.it

J. B. A. G. Haanen (✉)
Divisions of Medical Oncology and Molecular Oncology & Immunology, The Netherlands Cancer Institute, Amsterdam, The Netherlands
e-mail: j.haanen@nki.nl

© The Author(s) 2022
N. Kröger et al. (eds.), *The EBMT/EHA CAR-T Cell Handbook*,
https://doi.org/10.1007/978-3-030-94353-0_19

Similarly, the safety and antitumour activity of CAR-T cells targeting a variety of antigens, such as IL-13Rα2, epidermal growth factor receptor-vIII, and human epidermal growth factor receptor-2 (HER2), have been assessed in patients with glioblastoma multiforme (GBM). Infusion of second-generation CD28ζ HER2-specific CAR-modified virus-specific T cells was well tolerated, with no dose-limiting toxic effects, and led to clinical benefit; 1 patient showed a partial response (PR) lasting more than 9 months, and 7 patients had stable disease (SD) for several months (Ahmed et al. 2017). Other clinical trials have demonstrated the feasibility, safety, and clinical efficacy of second-generation EGFRvIII-specific and IL13BBζ–specific CAR-T cells (Brown et al. 2016) in patients with refractory GBM.

In gastrointestinal neoplasms, a clinical trial utilizing CEA CAR-T therapy in ten patients with metastatic colorectal cancer (CRC) resulted in SD in seven patients, without severe adverse events related to CAR-T therapy (Zhang et al. 2017). A previous case report of HER2-specific cell therapy for CRC using third generation CAR-T cells caused fatal acute respiratory distress syndrome due to recognition of lung epithelial cells expressing low levels of HER2 (Morgan et al. 2010). A phase I study of second-generation CAR-T cells targeting HER2 was conducted in 11 patients with advanced biliary tract cancer or pancreatic cancer. A 4.5-month partial response was observed, and 5 subjects achieved stable disease. Toxicity was manageable, with grade 3 fever and one patient showing elevation of liver enzymes as CAR-T-related adverse events; one episode of reversible severe upper gastrointestinal haemorrhage occurred in a patient with gastric involvement 11 days after the HER2 CAR-T- cell infusion, and 2 cases of grade 1–2 delayed fever accompanied by increases in C-reactive protein and interleukin-6 were observed (Feng et al. 2018). Epidermal growth factor receptor (EGFR) and CD133-specific CAR-T sequential immunotherapy were employed by the same group in a patient with advanced unresectable/metastatic cholangiocarcinoma (CCA), resulting in a PR lasting more than 12 months; however, slight liver toxicity secondary to EGFR CAR-T therapy and epidermal and endothelial damage due to CD133-specific CAR-T immunotherapy was observed.

Similar to these experiences, second-generation HER2-specific CAR-T cells, used in a phase I clinical trial conducted on 19 patients with refractory HER2-positive sarcoma, induced SD lasting from 12 weeks to 14 months in 4 of the evaluable patients (Ahmed et al. 2015).

Investigators at the University of Pennsylvania explored an approach based on mRNA-transduced CAR-T cells that target mesothelin (meso CAR-T) in patients with advanced malignant pleural mesothelioma (MPM) or advanced pancreatic cancer. In the first two patients reported, meso CAR-T cells showed some antitumour activity in vivo in the absence of distinct toxicities (Beatty et al. 2014). Second-generation CAR-T cells specific for EGFR were employed in a phase I study to treat 11 patients with advanced non-small-cell lung cancer (NSCLC), resulting in 2 PR cases and 5 SD cases, lasting from 2 to 8 months, with limited adverse events, including skin toxicity, nausea, vomiting, dyspnoea, and hypotension (Feng et al. 2016).

A few phase I studies and case series have reported CAR-T cell treatment for other solid tumours, such as melanoma, breast cancer, renal cell carcinoma, prostate cancer, and ovarian and seminal vesicle cancer (reviewed Fucà et al. 2020).

Various toxicities were observed after CAR-T cell infusion for treatment of solid tumours. In the setting of haematologic malignancies, cytokine release syndrome (CRS) is a frequent, potentially severe adverse event following CAR-T cell therapy. However, CRS, as well as the neurological toxicity (ICAN) sometimes observed in the haematologic setting, has not yet become a common event after CAR-T cell therapy for solid tumours, perhaps because of the lower tumour load. Conversely, CAR-T cells trials conducted in solid tumour cohorts showed critical, unexpected on-target, off-tumour toxicities resulting from the recognition by CAR-T cells of tumour antigens expressed on healthy tissues (Morgan et al. 2010; Lamers et al. 2013). Targeting tumour-specific antigens appears to result in fewer off-tumour effects, but whether these CAR-T cells have promising clinical efficacy remains to be seen, and many trials are still ongoing. Strategies to increase tumour selectivity while sparing healthy tissues are being evaluated to control on-target off-tumour toxicity.

Despite novel genetic engineering techniques and combinatorial approaches to counteract biological barriers, tumour heterogeneity, and the immunosuppressive properties of the tumour microenvironment, targeting solid tumours with CAR-T cells in the clinical setting remains challenging. Therefore, T cell therapy, alone or in combination with immune checkpoint inhibitors or other agents targeting either the cancer cell or the tumour environment, will likely play a role in improving cancer treatment outcomes (Apetoh et al. 2015). Designing and selecting the most appropriate clinical trials or settings to rapidly identify combinatorial approaches that are efficacious in different patient populations and identifying patients who will best benefit from immune checkpoint inhibitors alone (Chalabi et al. 2020) or from the addition of other targeted immunotherapies will be the most pressing need for the future success of CAR immunotherapy in solid cancer.

Key Points
- CAR-T therapy is under development for many solid cancer types, but important breakthroughs have not yet been achieved.
- Tumour heterogeneity, the immunosuppressive tumour microenvironment, and other barriers are hurdles that must be overcome before CAR-T cells can be effective against solid cancers.
- The field may benefit from network models for CAR-T cell production in academic centres.

References

Ahmed N, Brawley VS, Hegde M, et al. Human epidermal growth factor receptor 2 (HER2)-specific chimeric antigen receptor-modified T cells for the immunotherapy of HER2-positive sarcoma. J Clin Oncol. 2015;20(33):1688–96.

Ahmed N, Brawley V, Hegde M, et al. HER2-specific chimeric antigen receptor-modified virus-specific T cells for progressive glioblastoma: a phase 1 dose-escalation trial. JAMA Oncol. 2017;3:1094–101.

Apetoh L, Ladoire S, Coukos G, et al. Combining immunotherapy and anticancer agents: the right path to achieve cancer cure? Ann Oncol. 2015;26:1813–23.

Beatty GL, Haas AR, Maus MV, et al. Mesothelin-specific chimeric antigen receptor mRNA-engineered T cells induce anti-tumor activity in solid malignancies. Cancer Immunol Res. 2014;2:112–20.

Brown C, Alizadeh D, Starr R, et al. Regression of glioblastoma after chimeric antigen receptor T-cell therapy. N Engl J Med. 2016;375:2561–9.

Chalabi M, Fanchi LF, Dijkstra KK, et al. Neoadjuvant immunotherapy leads to pathological responses in MMR-proficient and MMR-deficient early-stage colon cancers. Nat Med. 2020;26:566–76.

Comoli P, Chabannon C, Koehl U, Lanza F, Urbano-Ispizua A, Hudecek M, Ruggeri A, Secondino S, Bonini C, Pedrazzoli P. Development of adaptive immune effector therapies in solid tumors. Ann Oncol. 2019;30:1740–50.

Feng K, Guo Y, Dai H, et al. Chimeric antigen receptor-modified T cells for the immunotherapy of patients with EGFR expressing advanced relapsed/refractory non-small cell lung cancer. Sci China Life Sci. 2016;59:468–79.

Feng K, Liu Y, Guo Y, Qiu J, Wu Z, Dai H, et al. Phase I study of chimeric antigen receptor modified T cells in treating HER2-positive advanced biliary tract cancers and pancreatic cancers. Protein Cell. 2018;9:838–47.

Fucà G, Reppel L, Landoni E, Savoldo B, Dotti G. Enhancing chimeric antigen receptor T-cell efficacy in solid tumors. Clin Cancer Res. 2020;26:2444–51.

Heczey A, Courtney AN, Montalbano A, Robinson S, Liu K, Li M, Ghatwai N, Dakhova O, Liu B, Raveh-Sadka T, Chauvin-Fleurence CN, Xu X, Ngai H, Di Pierro EJ, Savoldo B, Dotti G, Metelitsa LS. Anti-GD2 CAR-NKT cells in patients with relapsed or refractory neuroblastoma: an interim analysis. Nat Med. 2020;26:1686–90.

Lamers CH, Sleijfer S, van Steenbergen S, et al. Treatment of metastatic renal cell carcinoma with CAIX CAR-engineered T cells: clinical evaluation and management of on-target toxicity. Mol Ther. 2013;21:904–12.

Morgan RA, Yang JC, Kitano M, Dudley ME, Laurencot CM, Rosenberg SA. Case report of a serious adverse event following the administration of T cells transduced with a chimeric antigen receptor recognizing ERBB2. Mol Ther. 2010;18:843–51.

Pule M, Savoldo B, Myers GD, et al. Virus-specific T cells engineered to coexpress tumor-specific receptors: persistence and antitumor activity in individuals with neuroblastoma. Nat Med. 2008;14:1264–70.

Zhang C, Wang Z, Yang Z, et al. Phase I escalating-dose trial of CAR-T therapy targeting CEA(+) metastatic colorectal cancers. Mol Ther. 2017;25:1248–58.

Part IV

Clinical Management of Patients Treated with CAR-T Cells

Nicolas Boissel and Fabio Ciceri

Bridging therapy can be given after leukapheresis and before lymphodepletion during CAR-T cell manufacturing. The primary goal of bridging therapies is to prevent uncontrolled progression of the underlying disease during the manufacturing period before CAR-T cell infusion. Several studies indicate that a high tumour burden is associated with an increased risk of complications after CAR-T cell infusion (Cohen et al. 2019). Therefore, controlling the disease and even possibly decreasing the tumour burden is critical during the manufacturing period. The choice of bridging therapies is essential for the success of the procedure.

Clinical trials of CD19 CAR-T therapy in B-ALL reproducibly report high rates of patient dropout after enrolment due to disease progression or treatment-related complications (Park et al. 2018; Maude et al. 2018). For example, among 75 patients who received a CAR-T infusion in the ELIANA study, 65 (87%) were treated with bridging chemotherapy between enrolment and infusion, and 10 out of 92 patients enrolled in the trial could not be infused due to significant adverse events or death (Maude et al. 2018). The rate of adult patients infused in the Memorial Sloan Kettering (MSKCC) experience was 65% (54/83, 65%) of enrolled patients, mostly due to disease progression and death (Park et al. 2018). This reflects the challenges in clinical management during the 3–6-week period necessary for autologous CAR-T cell preparation (the bridging period).

N. Boissel
URP-3518, Institut de Recherche Saint-Louis, Université de Paris, Paris, France

Service d'Hématologie Adolescents et Jeunes Adultes, Assistance Publique des Hôpitaux de Paris, Paris, France
e-mail: nicolas.boissel@aphp.fr

F. Ciceri (✉)
Vita-Salute San Raffaele University, Milan, Italy

Hematology and Bone Marrow Transplantation Unit, IRCCS San Raffaele Hospital, Milan, Italy
e-mail: ciceri.fabio@hsr.it

© The Author(s) 2022
N. Kröger et al. (eds.), *The EBMT/EHA CAR-T Cell Handbook*,
https://doi.org/10.1007/978-3-030-94353-0_20

Given that CD19 CAR-T therapies are currently indicated for relapsed/refractory B-ALL patients who have already been exposed to one or more lines of potentially effective therapies, often including combinations of several agents, and that these patients often require therapeutic intervention against rapidly progressive disease or a high tumour burden, the choice of the better approach is not trivial.

Several bridging therapy options now exist, including high-intensity chemotherapy, targeted agents (e.g., TKIs), immunotherapies (e.g., CD-19 or CD22-directed), and low-intensity approaches (e.g., vincristine, 6-MP, steroids, thioguanine, etc.). Each approach has pros and cons. For example, high-intensity chemotherapy might be too toxic to allow treatment with CAR-T cells to proceed, while low-intensity approaches might fail in terms of tumour burden reduction.

In addition, treatment with CD19-directed therapies, such as the bispecific T cell engager blinatumomab, might have an impact on the efficacy of subsequent CD19 CAR-T cell therapy (Pillai et al. 2019), and common mechanisms of tumour escape to CD19-directed therapies have now been reported (Boissel 2021). Blinatumomab use was an exclusion criterion from the ELIANA trial (Maude et al. 2018), while it was allowed for patients participating in other similar trials. In the expanded access program for tisagenlecleucel, the overall response rate in patients with prior blinatumomab treatment was 67% versus 90% in other patients (Baruchel et al. 2020). However, no univocal data on this important salvage option are available in this setting.

In a recent study, the Memorial Sloan Kettering group reviewed different bridging strategies and outcomes for all patients enrolled in a single-centre, phase 1 trial of CD19-specific CAR-T cells for R/R adult ALL (ClinicalTrials.gov NCT01044069) (Perica et al. 2021). They observed that reductions in disease burden during the bridging period are associated with favourable outcomes after CAR-T therapy and thus suggest that optimal strategies to reduce disease burden during bridging are warranted. They proposed a bridging strategy based on disease burden at the time of the CAR-T therapy decision. They recommended low-intensity therapy for patients with a low tumour burden, low-intensity chemotherapy, or targeted therapy (e.g., inotuzumab) for patients with a high disease burden who are chemorefractory (e.g., partial or short response to prior line of chemotherapy) and unlikely to benefit from high-intensity bridging, and a careful evaluation of the risks and benefits of high- vs. low-intensity therapy for patients with high disease burden with expected chemosensitivity (e.g., limited prior chemotherapy exposure, late relapse, or sensitivity to the last line). In fact, not surprisingly, the study showed an increased rate of infections during the bridging period in the high-intensity chemotherapy group.

In conclusion, tumour burden, patient comorbidities, and disease characteristics should tailor the choice of the optimal bridging therapy. The goal of this therapy is not complete disease eradication per se but reduction of tumour burden, preserving the patient in good clinical condition for CAR-T cell infusion. The benefits of tumour burden reduction may be twofold, with (1) a reduction in the early risk of adverse events, including cytokine release syndrome and (2) a better outcome after CAR-T cell therapy. Although the role of B-cell-directed therapies should be further and carefully investigated in this setting, mainly to exclude possible interference with CAR-T cell expansion or activity, targeted and low-intensity approaches could be instrumental for this objective. Conversely, high-intensity chemotherapy should be limited to those cases in which the benefit and the probability of achieving a rapid tumour load reduction overcome the risk of infection or another toxic event in the context of a CAR-T-oriented strategy.

Key Point
- Disease control is necessary before CAR-T cell infusion.

References

Baruchel A, Krueger J, Balduzzi A, et al. Tisagenlecleucel for pediatric/young adults with relapsed/refractory acute lymphoblastic leukemia: preliminary report on B2001X study focusing on prior exposure to blinatumomab and inotuzumab. J Clin Oncol. 2020;38(15 Suppl):10518.

Boissel N. ALL in escape room. Blood. 2021;137(4):432–4.

Cohen AD, Garfall AL, Stadtmauer EA, et al. B cell maturation antigen-specific CAR-T cells are clinically active in multiple myeloma. J Clin Invest. 2019;129(6):2210–21.

Maude SL, Laetsch TW, Buechner J, Rives S, Boyer M, Bittencourt H, et al. Tisagenlecleucel in children and young adults with B-cell lymphoblastic leukemia. N Engl J Med. 2018;378:439–48.

Park JH, Rivière I, Gonen M, et al. Long-term follow-up of CD19 CAR-therapy in acute lymphoblastic leukemia. N Engl J Med. 2018;378:449–59.

Perica K, Flynn J, Curran KJ, et al. Impact of bridging chemotherapy on clinical outcome of CD19 CAR-T therapy in adult acute lymphoblastic leukemia. Leukemia. 2021;35(11):3268–71.

Pillai V, Muralidharan K, Meng W, et al. CAR-T cell therapy is effective for CD19-dim B-lymphoblastic leukemia but is impacted by prior blinatumomab therapy. Blood Adv. 2019;3:3539–49.

Further Reading

Anagnostou T, Riaz IB, Hashmiet SK, et al. Anti-CD19 chimeric antigen receptor T-cell therapy in acute lymphocytic leukaemia: a systematic review and metaanalysis. Lancet Haematol. 2020;7:e816–26.

Brentjens RJ, Rivière I, Park JH, et al. Safety and persistence of adoptively transferred autologous CD19-targeted T cells in patients with relapsed or chemotherapy refractory B-cell leukemias. Blood. 2011;118:4817–28.

Davila ML, Riviere I, Wang X, et al. Efficacy and toxicity management of 19-28z CAR-T cell therapy in B cell acute lymphoblastic leukemia. Sci Transl Med. 2014;6:224ra25.

Lee DW, Kochenderfer JN, Stetler-Stevenson M, et al. T cells expressing CD19 chimeric antigen receptors for acute lymphoblastic leukaemia in children and young adults: a phase 1 dose-escalation trial. Lancet. 2015;385:517–28.

Maude SL, Frey N, Shaw PA, et al. Chimeric antigen receptor T cells for sustained remissions in leukemia. N Engl J Med. 2014;371:1507–17.

Bridging to CAR-T Cells in Children, Adolescents, and Young Adults with ALL

21

André Baruchel

The Importance of the Bridge

Leukapheresis can be performed in most patients, including infants, but not all patients will receive autologous CAR-T cells. The ELIANA trial can be taken as an example to help understand the issues: 97 patients were successfully screened and enrolled, but only 79 of them finally made it to the infusion. Of the remaining 18 patients, 10 died or experienced an AE during the manufacturing time, and 8 patients had issues with the manufacturing process (Grupp et al. 2018).

Contrary to what is expected prior to allogeneic haematopoietic cell transplantation (allo-HCT), the role of an optimal bridging therapy is not to obtain the lowest residual disease but only a reduction or stabilization of tumour burden, bringing the patient to the CAR-T cell infusion in good clinical condition.

Some facts are to recall:

- The interval between apheresis and infusion is highly variable and during clinical trials can range between 3 weeks and 3 months. With the approved commercial product tisagenlecleucel, the interval is now in the 3–4-week range. Of note, manufacturing could be shorter in academic closed systems using fresh cells and decentralized manufacturing.
- Many variables can indeed influence the final interval:
  - Cryopreservation to shipping: time can be lost, being influenced by manufacturing slots.
  - Manufacturing site: USA vs. EU.

A. Baruchel (✉)
Université de Paris et EA 3518 Institut de Recherche Saint-Louis, Paris, France

Service d'Hémato-Immunologie Pédiatrique, Hôpital Universitaire Robert Debré (APHP), Paris, France
e-mail: andre.baruchel@rdb.aphp.fr

© The Author(s) 2022
N. Kröger et al. (eds.), *The EBMT/EHA CAR-T Cell Handbook*,
https://doi.org/10.1007/978-3-030-94353-0_21

- Availability of the cell therapy lab to receive the apheresis product and then the common availability of the same lab and the pharmacists to receive the "drug".
- Availability of a room in the clinical department and the possibility that the patient can be admitted to the ICU in the case of complications, which can be an issue in the current pandemic.
- Of utmost importance are the course of the disease and the clinical status, with the main risks being disease progression, occurrence of infection (fungal diseases in particular) in these heavily pretreated patients and other SAEs linked to chemo/immunotherapies (e.g., inotuzumab).

Thus, the « art of bridging » includes the following steps:

- Selecting the best chemotherapy requires integrating the disease biology, previous disease sensitivity to treatment and the tolerance history of the patient. There is no « one size fits all » here.
- Aiming to undergo lymphodepletion plus infusion without too much disease as a way to decrease the incidence of CRS and increase the final outcome.
- Monitoring a patient who is not completely under your control: close collaboration and numerous contacts (at least 2/week) with the referring centre are mandatory.

Examples of possible choices are found in Table 21.1.

Table 21.1 Possible bridging therapies on the road to CAR-T cell therapy according to tumour burden and disease localization and kinetics[a]

No treatment: smouldering disease
Low-intensity chemotherapy: low disease burden and/or slowly progressing ALL • Weekly vincristine (VCR) with oral 6MP and methotrexate (MTX). • Weekly VCR plus dexamethasone (DEX) 6 mg/m^2 2 days/week.
Intermediate-intensity chemotherapy: disease burden and/or progressing ALL • Consolidation « IB » (6MP, cytarabine, cyclophosphamide). • Weekly VCR plus DEX, bortezomib, asparaginase.
High-intensity chemotherapy: aggressive disease or EMD[b] • High-dose (HD) cytarabine, VP16-cyclophosphamide, hyper CVAD. • High-dose MTX if CNS involvement.
Very high-intensity chemotherapy for rapidly progressing disease: • Sequential approach, e.g., HD cytarabine followed by LD.

[a] Targeted agents, such as TKIs, can be used in Ph+ ALL and ABL class fusion ALL in addition to low-intensity chemotherapy, for example
[b] EMD: extramedullary disease

Is There a Place for Immunotherapy?

- Accumulating data suggest that the use of CD19-oriented therapy (e.g., blinatumomab) prior to administration of CD19 CAR-T cells can be detrimental, particularly with the selection of CD19-negative clones (Pillai et al. 2019; Baruchel et al. 2020; Taraseviciute et al. 2020).
- Inotuzumab ozogamicin, an anti-CD22 therapy, can be used in patients with chemoresistant disease but can result in a high rate of negative MRD, sometimes with no remaining normal B cells, which could theoretically lead to an insufficient target level for adequate CAR-T cell expansion and persistence. In a recent clinical trial (Baruchel et al. 2020), this treatment was associated with a diminished EFS. Inotuzumab ozogamicin is also not recommended prior to the use of anti-CD22 CAR-T cells.

> **Key Points**
> - The aim of optimal bridging therapy is not to obtain the lowest residual disease possible but only to reduce or stabilize the tumour burden, bringing the patient to CAR-T cell infusion in good clinical condition.
> - There is no "one size fits all" in this area. Deep knowledge of disease biology, emerging targets, previous sensitivity to treatment, and the tolerance history of the patient are needed.

References

Baruchel A, Krueger J, Balduzzi A. Tisagenlecleucel for pediatric/young adult patients with relapsed/refractory b-cell acute lymphoblastic leukemia: preliminary report of B2001X focusing on prior exposure to blinatumomab and inotuzumab. EHA Library. 2020;294938:S118.

Grupp SA, Maude SL, Rives S, et al. Updated analysis of the efficacy and safety of tisagenlecleucel in pediatric and young adult patients with relapsed/refractory (r/r) acute lymphoblastic leukemia. Blood. 2018;132(Suppl 1):895.

Pillai V, Muralidharan K, Meng W, et al. CAR-T cell therapy is effective for CD19-dim B-lymphoblastic leukemia but is impacted by prior blinatumomab therapy. Blood Adv. 2019;3:3539–49.

Taraseviciute A, Steinberg SM, Myers RM, et al. Pre-CAR blinatumomab is associated with increased post-CD19 CAR relapse and decreased event free survival. Blood. 2020;136(Suppl 1):13–4.

Bridging Chemotherapy: Relapsed/Refractory Aggressive B-Cell Lymphoma

Catherine Thieblemont and Peter Borchmann

To Bridge or Not to Bridge in Relapsed and Refractory (R/R) Aggressive B-Cell Lymphoma?

The time interval between leukapheresis and CAR-T cell infusion is critical for many patients with R/R B-cell lymphoma and symptomatic disease that could be fatal if left untreated during the cell manufacturing period. Often, oncologists address this dilemma with bridging therapy (BT), which may include steroids, chemotherapy, targeted therapy, or radiation therapy.

However, the R/R DLBCL patients included in the ZUMA-1 trial that led to axi-cel approval were not allowed to receive BT other than dexamethasone (Neelapu et al. 2017). In contrast, the JULIET and TRANSCEND trials leading to approval of tisa-cel and liso-cel, respectively, allowed various treatments, including systemic therapy, radiation therapy, or both (Schuster et al. 2019; Locke et al. 2019; Abramson et al. 2020). In these latest trials, bridging therapy was used in 159 (59%) of 269 patients in TRANSCEND and 92% of patients in JULIET at the investigator's discretion. Importantly, patients receiving BT are likely to have more aggressive disease and, therefore, are more likely to have other risk factors for increased rates of cytokine release syndrome, neurological events, or both, such as an increased serum lactate dehydrogenase (LDH) level, increased sum of product diameter or higher

C. Thieblemont (✉)
Université de Paris, Paris, France

Hôpital Saint-Louis, Service d'Hémato-oncologie, DMU DHI, Assistance Publique des Hôpitaux de Paris, Paris, France
e-mail: catherine.thieblemont@aphp.fr

P. Borchmann
Department I of Internal Medicine, University Hospital of Cologne, Cologne, Germany
e-mail: peter.borchmann@uk-koeln.de

© The Author(s) 2022
N. Kröger et al. (eds.), *The EBMT/EHA CAR-T Cell Handbook*,
https://doi.org/10.1007/978-3-030-94353-0_22

total metabolic tumour burden (TMTV) before lymphodepleting chemotherapy, and increased baseline C-reactive protein level.

Up to 87% of patients treated with axi-cel or tisa-cel in real-world settings required BT (Nastoupil et al. 2020; Vercellino et al. 2020). However, in most patients, bridging therapy did not result in a lower tumour burden at the time of CAR-T cell reinfusion (Locke et al. 2019).

Which Bridging Therapy?

The time between leukapheresis and infusion may vary between the USA and Europe. In France, this duration of time was described to be approximately 50 days. The median number of treatment cycles during the bridge was two cycles (range, 1–4; IQR, 1–2). Bridging therapy consisted of various immunochemotherapy or chemotherapy regimens described as high-intensity BT and low-dose BT, including chemo-free regimens. Because of lymphoma progression, 31% received more than 1 line of bridging therapy. Table 22.1 describes different BT options.

The choice will be based on

1. Evaluation of the tumour mass and growth kinetics, including the LDH level, sum of product diameter, and/or TMTV;
2. The biology of the disease, including cell of origin;
3. The type of prior lines and refractoriness or sensitivity; and
4. Patient characteristics, including comorbidities and resilience.

Table 22.1 Possible bridging therapies

No treatment: asymptomatic disease without clinically relevant tumour mass or growth
Low-intensity treatment: low disease burden (For off-label drug use, please check the local requirements)
• Rituximab-dexamethasone
• Brentuximab vedotin
• Lenalidomide
• Radiotherapy
• Single agent chemotherapy, e.g., etoposide, gemcitabine, pixantrone
High-intensity treatment: aggressive disease
• Ifosfamide-VP16 with or without rituximab
• ICE (ifosfamide-carboplatinum-etoposide) with or without brentuximab vedotin or rituximab
• GEMOX (gemcitabine-oxaliplatin) with or without rituximab
• Polatuzumab-bendamustine-rituximab
Very high-intensity treatment for rapidly progressing disease
• High-dose melphalan with autologous stem cell support
• Hyperfractionated cyclophosphamide in combination regimens, e.g., hyperCVAD

Response Rate to Bridging Therapy and Subsequent CAR-T Cell Therapy

Across the clinical trials, objective responses were achieved across all subgroups, including in patients receiving bridging therapy (Locke et al. 2019). Durable responses were also seen in patients who received BT (Locke et al. 2019). However, in real life, early relapses were associated with high-intensity BT (Vercellino et al. 2020), correlated with a higher tumour burden and more rapidly progressive symptomatic disease at the time of selection. Similarly, Nastoupil and coworkers showed that among the patients who received axi-cel infusion, bridging therapy was not associated with OS but may have negatively affected PFS, particularly among those who received systemic BT. Intriguingly, patients who received bridging radiotherapy had superior PFS vs. patients who were bridged with systemic therapy, despite comparable baseline characteristics (Nastoupil et al. 2020).

Key Points
The decisions of whether to administer bridging therapy and which bridging therapy to choose require consideration of the following factors:

- Evaluation of **the lymphoma growth kinetics** based on measurement of the tumour volume at the time of apheresis, ideally measured by total metabolic tumour volume on an 18-FDG PET scan or bulk disease (>7.5 cm) or widespread disease (Ann Arbor III or IV) evaluated on a CT scan, and elevation of LDH levels above the upper normal value (UNV).
- Integration of the **biology of the tumour** with the possibility of choosing targeted therapies, such as therapy with a monoclonal antibody (anti-CD30, anti-CD20), BTK inhibitor or lenalidomide.
- **Close monitoring of the patient,** who may not be completely under your control: a close collaboration and numerous contacts (at least 1/week) with the referring centre is mandatory.
- **All treatments** can be used based on the growth kinetics and biology of the tumour, individual patient characteristics, and prior lines, with one goal: controlling the disease up to the time of CAR-T cell reinfusion.

References

Abramson JS, Palomba LM, Gordon LI, et al. Lisocabtagene maraleucel for patients with relapsed or refractory large B-cell lymphomas (TRANSCEND NHL 001): a multicentre seamless design study. Lancet. 2020;396(10254):839–52.

Locke F, Ghobadi A, Jacobson C, et al. Long-term safety and activity of axicabtagene ciloleucel in refractory large B-cell lymphoma (ZUMA-1): a single-arm, multicentre, phase 1-2 trial. Lancet Oncol. 2019;20(1):31–42.

Nastoupil LJ, Jain MD, Feng L, et al. Standard-of-care axicabtagene ciloleucel for relapsed or refractory large B-cell lymphoma: results from the US Lymphoma CAR-T Consortium. J Clin Oncol. 2020;38(27):3119–28.

Neelapu S, Locke F, Bartlett N, et al. Axicabtagene ciloleucel CAR-T cell therapy in refractory large B-cell lymphoma. N Engl J Med. 2017;377(26):2531–44.

Schuster S, Bishop M, Tam C, et al. JULIET Investigators. Tisagenlecleucel in adult relapsed or refractory diffuse large B-cell lymphoma. N Engl J Med. 2019;380(1):45–56.

Vercellino L, Di Blasi R, Kanoun S, et al. Predictive factors of early progression after CAR-T cell therapy in relapsed/refractory diffuse large B-cell lymphoma. Blood Adv. 2020;4(22):5607–15.

Bridging Chemotherapy: Follicular Lymphoma, Mantle Cell Lymphoma, and CLL

23

Nico Gagelmann, John Gribben ⓘ, and Nicolaus Kröger ⓘ

While lisocabtagene maraleucel (liso-cel) is the only product that is specifically approved to treat grade 3B follicular lymphoma (FL), specifically in aggressive lymphoma indications, to date, axi-cel is the first and only approved CAR-T product for indolent NHL.

ZUMA-5 is a phase 2 study of axi-cel in patients with indolent NHL (including FL and marginal zone lymphoma (MZL)) treated with two or more prior lines of systemic therapy, with prior exposure to both an alkylating agent and anti-CD20 therapy (Jacobson et al. 2021). Of the 104 patients evaluable for efficacy, the ORR was 92% and the CR was 76%. For the 84 patients with FL, the ORR was 95% (CR 80%), and for the 20 patients with MZL, the ORR was 85% (CR 60%). No differences between prior treatments were noted, while to date, specific analyses according to bridging have not yet been presented. In the ELARA trial on tisa-cel in FL, 97 patients received treatment (median follow-up time, 10.6 months) (Schuster et al. 2021). The median number of prior therapies was 4 (range, 2–13); 78% of patients were refractory to their last treatment (76% to any ≥2 prior regimens) and 60% progressed within 2 years of initial anti-CD20-containing treatment. The CR rate was 66%, and the ORR was 86%, which was comparable among key subgroups, including bridging.

However, notably, indolent NHL is a chronic disease that can relapse after years of remission. Although the rates of continued CR and PFS at 12 months reported in ZUMA-5 are encouraging, a longer follow-up time is needed to identify patients who benefit the most from certain treatment sequences.

N. Gagelmann · N. Kröger (✉)
Department of Stem Cell Transplantation, University Medical Center Hamburg-Eppendorf, Hamburg, Germany
e-mail: n.gagelmann@uke.de; n.kroeger@uke.de

J. Gribben
Bart's Cancer Institute, Queen Mary University of London, London, UK
e-mail: j.gribben@qmul.ac.uk

Among relapsed or refractory mantle cell lymphoma patients receiving KTE-X19 CAR-T therapy (Wang et al. 2020), a total of 25 patients (37% of the total cohort) received bridging therapy with ibrutinib (14 patients), acalabrutinib (5), dexamethasone (12), or methylprednisolone (2). The majority of the patients who had assessments both before and after bridging therapy showed an increase in the median tumour burden after the receipt of bridging therapy. Response rates were similar regardless of exposure to bridging therapy, but ongoing responses seemed to be higher in patients without bridging therapy (67% vs. 38%).

With regard to chronic lymphocytic leukaemia, the TRANSCEND CLL 004 study of liso-cel included patients with standard or high-risk features treated with ≥ 3 or ≥ 2 prior therapies (Siddiqi et al. 2021), respectively, including Bruton kinase inhibitors. A total of 17 patients (74%) received bridging therapy during liso-cel manufacturing, and response rates were consistent, with 82% and 45% achieving overall and complete responses, respectively. Safety and efficacy were similar between treatment groups. Another small study even suggested the feasibility of concurrent ibrutinib with CD19 CAR-T therapy (Gauthier et al. 2020), but the population overall is still limited, and studies are ongoing.

> **Key Points**
> - Limited evidence on the role of bridging therapy in FL and indolent lymphoma.
> - Systemic therapy led to worse outcomes across lymphoma types, but the reasons are elusive.
> - Bendamustine should be avoided whenever possible.
> - The association between tumour volume before and after bridging therapy and the overall response after CAR-T cell therapy is still unclear in mantle cell lymphoma.
> - Bridging therapy in CLL with BTKi seems feasible.

References

Gauthier J, Hirayama AV, Purushe J, et al. Feasibility and efficacy of CD19-targeted CAR-T cells with concurrent ibrutinib for CLL after ibrutinib failure. Blood. 2020;135:1650–60.

Jacobson CA, Chavez JC, Sehgal AR, et al. Outcomes in ZUMA-5 with axicabtagene ciloleucel in patients with relapsed/refractory indolent non-Hodgkin lymphoma who had the high-risk feature of early progression after first chemoimmunotherapy. Abstract #S213. Presented at the EHA2021 Virtual Congress 2021 Jun 9.

Schuster SJ, Dickinson MJ, Dreyling MH, et al. Efficacy and safety of tisagenlecleucel (Tisa-cel) in adult patients (Pts) with relapsed/refractory follicular lymphoma (r/r FL): primary analysis of the phase 2 Elara trial. J Clin Oncol. 2021;39:7508.

Siddiqi T, Soumerai JD, Dorritie KA, et al. Phase 1 TRANSCEND CLL 004 study of lisocabtagene maraleucel in patients with relapsed/refractory CLL or SLL. Blood. 2021;

Wang M, Munoz J, Goy A, et al. KTE-X19 CAR-T cell therapy in relapsed or refractory mantle-cell lymphoma. N Engl J Med. 2020;382:1331–42.

Bridging Chemotherapy: Multiple Myeloma

24

Salomon Manier, Artur Jurczyszyn, and David H. Vesole

Should All MM Patients Receive Bridging Therapy?

In the phase 2 KarMMa study, 88% of the patients received bridging therapy with only a 5% response (Munshi et al. 2021). In the CARTITUDE 1 trial, 75% of the patients received bridging therapy, with a reduction in tumour burden observed in 34% of the patients prior to cilta-cel infusion, but no patients achieved a CR or better while on bridging therapy (Madduri et al. 2019). Bridging therapy is recommended for virtually all patients. An exception can be discussed for patients with slowly progressive disease, who may not need to receive bridging therapy after leukapheresis; however, this strategy exposes them to a risk of rapid progression later during the manufacturing period. In the future, with allogeneic CAR-T cells, bridging therapy will likely not be necessary because the time between patient inclusion and CAR-T cell infusion is much reduced.

S. Manier (✉)
Department of Hematology, Lille University, CHU Lille, Lille, France
e-mail: Salomon.MANIER@chru-lille.fr

A. Jurczyszyn
Plasma Cell Dyscrasia Center, Department of Hematology, Jagiellonian University Medical College, Krakow, Poland
e-mail: mmjurczy@cyf-kr.edu.pl

D. H. Vesole
Hackensack Meridian School of Medicine, Hackensack, NJ, USA
e-mail: David.Vesole@hmhn.org

Timeframe to Use Bridging Treatments

Bridging therapy can be started immediately after leukapheresis. Most clinical trials do not permit the use of any bridging therapy within 2 weeks prior to lymphodepletion to allow for haematologic recovery and to prevent any interaction between the drugs and the CAR-T cells (Munshi et al. 2021; Madduri et al. 2019).

Choice of Treatment

Several clinical trials allow only agents to which the patients have been previously exposed. However, this strategy can limit the efficacy of bridging therapy if patients are refractory to their previous treatments. Therefore, bridging therapies are typically personalized to each patient according to previous lines of treatment, disease characteristics, and pre-existing toxicities. All treatments can be considered for bridging therapy, including proteasome inhibitors, immunomodulatory drugs, anti-CD38 antibodies, targeted therapies, and conventional chemotherapies, with the exception of anti-BCMA targeting therapies in the case of BCMA-targeting CAR-T cells to avoid saturation of antigens. The risk of prolonged cytopenia and the risk of infection should also be taken into account when considering conventional chemotherapies. Involved field radiation therapy has been safely used during bridging (Manjunath et al. 2020).

> **Key Points**
> - Virtually all patients should receive bridging therapy to prevent rapid progression of the disease during the manufacturing period.
> - All treatments can be used with the exception of anti-BCMA therapies in the case of BCMA-targeting CAR-T cells.

References

Madduri D, Usmani SZ, Jagannath S, et al. Results from CARTITUDE-1: a phase 1b/2 study of JNJ-4528, a CAR-T cell therapy directed against B-cell maturation antigen (BCMA), in patients with relapsed and/or refractory multiple myeloma (R/R MM). Blood. 2019;134(Suppl 1):577.

Manjunath SH, Cohen AD, Arscott WT, Maity A, Plastaras JP, Paydar I. Is Bridging Radiation (RT) Safe with B Cell Maturation Antigen–targeting Chimeric Antigenic Receptor T Cells (CART-BCMA) Therapy? ASTRO. 2020;1104

Munshi NC, Anderson LD Jr, Shah N, et al. Idecabtagene vicleucel in relapsed and refractory multiple myeloma. N Engl J Med. 2021;384(8):705–16.

Lymphodepleting Conditioning Regimens

25

Mohamad Mohty and Monique C. Minnema

Lymphodepleting conditioning regimens are essential for the success of CAR-T cell treatment. Their importance in the proliferation and persistence of CAR-T cells has become clearer in the recent years. The suggested mechanisms are described in Table 25.1 and include the effects on immune cells and cytokines, creating an environment for optimal functioning and increasing the peak of expansion of the infused CAR-T cells (Neelapu 2019).

The addition of fludarabine to cyclophosphamide has been important in increasing the efficacy of CAR-T cell treatment and is currently the most commonly used combination (Turtle et al. 2016). In the applied conditioning regimens, the dosing of fludarabine is relatively consistent, with the use of 25–30 mg/m², given on 3 sequential days, but the dosing of cyclophosphamide differs in days and intensity. A "higher intensity" cyclophosphamide dosing regimen seems to be preferred (Hirayama et al. 2019). However, even with the best lymphodepletion regimen, some patients fail to develop a favourable cytokine profile, suggesting that the host biological response to lymphodepletion chemotherapy is important (Hirayama et al. 2019). Most conditioning regimens can be given on an outpatient basis.

In Hodgkin lymphoma treated with anti-CD30 CAR-T cells, bendamustine has been used as conditioning regimen, but in this disease, the addition of fludarabine to the regimen has also been shown to increase antitumour responses. Whether an even more intensive regimen is needed in solid tumours is currently unknown.

M. Mohty (✉)
Sorbonne University, Saint-Antoine Hospital, Paris, France
e-mail: mohamad.mohty@inserm.fr

M. C. Minnema
Department of Hematology, University Medical Center Utrecht, University Utrecht, Utrecht, The Netherlands
e-mail: M.C.Minnema@umcutrecht.nl

© The Author(s) 2022
N. Kröger et al. (eds.), *The EBMT/EHA CAR-T Cell Handbook*,
https://doi.org/10.1007/978-3-030-94353-0_25

Table 25.1 Adapted from Neelapu (2019)

Effects of a conditioning regimen	
Lymphodepletion	Lowers total NK, B, and T cells
Fewer anti-CAR-T cell immune responses	Reduces anti-transgene immune reactions
Eradication of immune suppressor cells	Tregs and MDSCs
Modulation of tumour suppressive effects	Lowers IDO expression, increases levels of costimulatory molecules
Elimination of homeostatic cytokine sink	Increases IL-2, IL-7, IL-15, and MCP-1 expression levels
Increased expansion, function, and persistence of CAR-T cells	Better and durable tumour responses

Tregs regulatory T cells, *MDSCs* myeloid-derived suppressor cells, *IDO* indoleamine deoxygenase, *MCP-1* monocyte chemoattractant protein-1

The timing of the conditioning regimen is typically within a week before the planned infusion, with a minimum of 2 resting days to avoid a negative impact of chemotherapy on the infused cells. If, after the start of the conditioning regimen, the patient cannot receive CAR-T cells, most protocols allow a waiting time of 2–4 weeks before a new conditioning regimen must be started. In other protocols, conditioning regimens are not given if the absolute lymphocyte count is below 200 cells/µL.

The negative effects of conditioning regimens include pancytopenia and prolonged immune suppression and add to the enhanced risk of (viral) infections seen after CAR-T cell treatment. In addition, fludarabine can induce fever, neurotoxicity, cyclophosphamide haemorrhagic cystitis, and pericarditis, and both drugs may increase the risk of secondary malignancies.

Key Points
- An effective lymphodepleting regimen increases the proliferation and persistence of CAR-T cells.
- Fludarabine seems essential and is typically used with cyclophosphamide.

References

Hirayama AV, Gauthier J, Hay KA, et al. The response to lymphodepletion impacts PFS in patients with aggressive non-Hodgkin lymphoma treated with CD19 CAR-T cells. Blood. 2019;133:1876–87.

Neelapu SS. CAR-T efficacy: is conditioning the key? Blood. 2019;133:1799–800.

Turtle CJ, Hanafi L-A, Berger C, et al. Immunotherapy of non-Hodgkin's lymphoma with a defined ratio of CD8+ and CD4+ CD19-specific chimeric antigen receptor–modified T cells. Sci Transl Med. 2016;8:1–12.

Management of Cytokine Release Syndrome (CRS) and HLH

26

Francis Ayuk Ayuketang and Ulrich Jäger

Cytokine Release Syndrome (CRS)

Definition and Occurrence

Cytokine release syndrome (CRS) is caused by a rapid and mild to massive release of cytokines from immune cells involved in immune reactions, particularly after immunotherapy. The frequency and severity of CRS after CAR-T cell therapy varies between products (any grade: 37–93%, G3/4: 1–23%) (Neelapu et al. 2017; Schuster et al. 2019; Abramson et al. 2020).

Diagnosis

Clinical Symptoms, Laboratory Diagnosis, Differential Diagnosis, and Predictive Factors

CRS usually manifests with fever preceding or accompanied by general symptoms, such as malaise, headache, arthralgia, anorexia, rigours, and fatigue, and can rapidly progress to hypoxia, tachypnoea, tachycardia, hypotension, arrhythmia, culminating in shock cardiorespiratory organ dysfunction, and failure.

Although the diagnosis of CRS cannot be established or ruled out by laboratory diagnostics, they can be used to monitor organ dysfunction. CRS symptoms and laboratory findings closely mimic infection; therefore, infectious workup and

F. A. Ayuketang
Department of Stem Cell Transplantation, University Medical Center Hamburg, Hamburg, Germany
e-mail: ayuketang@uke.de

U. Jäger (✉)
Medical University of Vienna, Department of Medicine I, Division of Hematology and Hemostaseology, Vienna, Austria
e-mail: Ulrich.jaeger@meduniwien.ac.at

© The Author(s) 2022
N. Kröger et al. (eds.), *The EBMT/EHA CAR-T Cell Handbook*,
https://doi.org/10.1007/978-3-030-94353-0_26

treatment are of primary importance. Other relevant differential diagnoses include tumour lysis and progression of the underlying malignancy.

Prediction of CRS in an individual patient is not yes possible. However, some factors, such as high tumour burden and CAR-T cell dose, seem to be associated with a higher risk of CRS.

Management

Patients receiving CAR-T cells should be monitored continuously or at regular intervals for cardiovascular function and temperature. The first sign of CRS is usually fever. Mild CRS (G1) can be managed conservatively. All higher grades require intensive monitoring and intervention. Early use of tocilizumab and, in some cases, steroids is now recommended (Table 26.1) (Yakoub-Agha et al. 2020).

Table 26.1 Scoring of CRS (adapted from Yakoub-Agha et al. 2020)

CRS Parameter	Grad 1	Grad 2	Grad 3	Grad 4
Fever	Fever ≥38°C (not attributable to any other cause). In patients who have CRS then receive antipyretics or anticytokine therapy such as tocilizumab or steriods, fever is no longer required to grade subsequent CRS severity. In this case, CRS grading is driven by hypotension and/or hypoxia.			
Hypotension	None	Not requiring vasopressors	Requiring a vasopressor with or without vasopressin	Requiring multiple vasopressors (excluding vasopressin)
Hypoxia	None	Requiring low-flow oxygen (delivered at ≤ 6l/min)	Requiring high-flow oxygen (delivered at > 6l/min)	Requiring positive pressure (e.g. CPAP, BiPAP, intubation and mechanical ventilation)

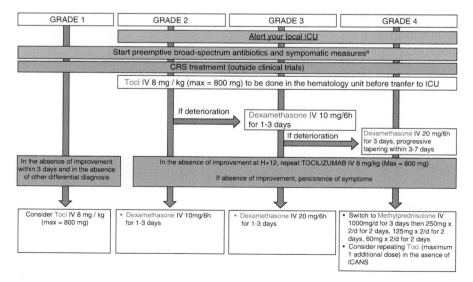

Fig. 26.1 Management of CRS—Modified according to EBMT recommendations

Monitoring: Patients with CRS 1 can be monitored on the regular ward or Intermediate Care ward, starting from G2, and admission to an ICU should be considered.

Supportive therapy consists of fluids and antipyretics. The use of vasopressors automatically marks higher grade CRS.

Anti-Cytokines

Tocilizumab is EMA and FDA approved for the treatment of CRS. Prophylactic, preemptive or risk-adapted use may reduce the risk of severe CRS without attenuating antitumour efficacy.

(Locke et al. 2017; Caimi et al. 2020; Gardner et al. 2019; Kadauke et al. 2021). Clinical trial data on the use of siltuximab and anakinra are still lacking.

Steroids

In contrast to initial clinical studies, short courses of steroids do not seem to have detrimental effects on CAR-T cell expansion and survival or clinical outcome.

Antibiotics

Because CRS cannot be decisively differentiated from infection, most centres administer antibiotic treatment in cases of neutropenic fever. However, the use of growth factors during the first few weeks should be restricted. GM-CSF is to be avoided.

sHLH/MAS

Secondary or reactive haemophagocytic lymphohistiocytosis (sHLH) is a life-threatening hyperinflammation syndrome that occurs in the context of allo-HCT, haematological malignancies, infection, and rheumatic or autoimmune disease and is characterized by hyperactive macrophages and lymphocytes, haemophagocytosis, and multiorgan damage (Carter et al. 2019; Neelapu et al. 2018; Sandler et al. 2020). The proposed diagnostic criteria are summarized in Table 26.2. Management of sHLH generally follows similar algorithms as that for severe CRS. In refractory patients, treatment may follow the management framework proposed by Mehta et al. (2020), with a key role for anakinra.

Table 26.2 Diagnostic criteria for HLA (adapted from Neelapu et al. 2018)

Diagnostik criteria for CAR-T cell mediated sHLA/MAS (Neelapu et al., 2018)	Adult HScore (Fardet et al., 2014): Respective scores are in brackets Produces a probability outcome; scores >169 are 93% sensitive and 86% specific for HLH	
Clinical	Clinical	
Grade ≥3 pulmonary oedema*	Fever	<38.4 (0); 38.4–39.4 (33); >39.4 (49)
	Hepatomegaly /	Neither (0); either hepatomegaly or splenomegaly (23); both (38)
	Immunosuppression	No (0); yes (18)
Labotarory	Laboratory	
Peak ferritin 10.000ng/ml during CRS and any 2 of the following	Ferritin, ng/mL	<2000 (0); 2000-6000 (35); >6000 (50)
Grade ≥3 increase in serum bilirubin, aspartate aminotransferase, or alanine aminotransferase levels*	Cytopenias >2 lineages	One lineage (0), two lineages (24), or three lineages (34)
Grade ≥3 oliguria or increase in serum creatinine levels*	Hypertriglyceridaemia, mmol	<1.5 (0); 1.5-4 (44); >4 (64)
Presence of haemophagocytosis in bone marrow or organs based on histopathological assessment of cell morphology and/or CD68 immunohistochemistry	Haemophagocytosis	No (0), yes (35)
*According to Common Terminology Criteria for Adverse Events (CTCAE) Version 4.0	Liver function tests, IU/L	AST<30 (0); >30 (19)
	Hypofibrinogenaemia, g/L	>2.5 (0); <2.5 (30)

Key Points
- Cytokine release syndrome is a frequent complication. However, severe CRS is rare if management is proactive.
- sHLH/MAS is a rare but severe complication that requires prompt recognition and intervention.

References

Abramson JS, Palomba ML, Gordon LI, et al. Lisocabtagene maraleucel for patients with relapsed or refractory large B-cell lymphomas (TRANSCEND NHL 001): a multicentre seamless design study. Lancet. 2020;396(10254):839–52.

Caimi PF, Sharma A, Rojas P, et al. CAR-T therapy for lymphoma with prophylactic tocilizumab: decreased rates of severe cytokine release syndrome without excessive neurologic toxicity. Blood. 2020;136:30–1. https://ash.confex.com/ash/2020/webprogram/Paper143114.html

Carter SJ, Tattersall RS, Ramanan AV. Macrophage activation syndrome in adults: recent advances in pathophysiology, diagnosis and treatment. Rheumatology (Oxford). 2019;58(1):5–17.

Gardner RA, Ceppi F, Rivers J, et al. Preemptive mitigation of CD19 CAR-T cell cytokine release syndrome without attenuation of antileukemic efficacy. Blood. 2019;134(24):2149–58.

Kadauke S, Myers RM, Li Y, et al. Risk-adapted preemptive tocilizumab to prevent severe cytokine release syndrome after CTL019 for pediatric B-cell acute lymphoblastic leukemia: a prospective clinical trial. J Clin Oncol. 2021;39(8):920–30.

Locke FL, Neelapu SS, Bartlett NL, et al. Preliminary results of prophylactic Tocilizumab after axicabtagene ciloleucel (axi-cel; KTE-C19) treatment for patients with refractory, aggressive non-Hodgkin lymphoma (NHL). Blood. 2017;130(Supplement 1):1547.

Mehta P, Cron RQ, Hartwell J, Manson JJ, Tattersall RS. Silencing the cytokine storm: the use of intravenous anakinra in haemophagocytic lymphohistiocytosis or macrophage activation syndrome. Lancet Rheumatol. 2020;2(6):e358–67.

Neelapu SS, Locke FL, Bartlett NL, et al. Axicabtagene Ciloleucel CAR-T cell therapy in refractory large B-cell lymphoma. N Engl J Med. 2017;377(26):2531–44.

Neelapu SS, Tummala S, Kebriaei P, et al. Chimeric antigen receptor T-cell therapy – assessment and management of toxicities. Nat Rev Clin Oncol. 2018;15(1):47–62.

Sandler RD, Carter S, Kaur H, Francis S, Tattersall RS, Snowden JA. Haemophagocytic lymphohistiocytosis (HLH) following allogeneic haematopoietic stem cell transplantation (HSCT)-time to reappraise with modern diagnostic and treatment strategies? Bone Marrow Transplant. 2020;55(2):307–16.

Schuster SJ, Bishop MR, Tam CS, et al. Tisagenlecleucel in adult relapsed or refractory diffuse large B-cell lymphoma. N Engl J Med. 2019;380(1):45–56.

Yakoub-Agha I, Chabannon C, Bader P, et al. Management of adults and children undergoing chimeric antigen receptor T-cell therapy: best practice recommendations of the European Society for Blood and Marrow Transplantation (EBMT) and the joint accreditation committee of ISCT and EBMT (JACIE). Haematologica. 2020;105(2):297–316.

Management of Immune Effector Cell-Associated Neurotoxicity Syndrome (ICANS)

27

Jeremy H. Rees

A common and challenging side effect associated with CAR-T cell therapy is immune cell-associated neurotoxicity syndrome (ICANS), which occurs in 20–60% of patients, of whom 12–30% have severe ($\geq$ grade 3) symptoms.

The underlying mechanism driving the syndrome is not fully understood, but there is evidence for the release of inflammatory cytokines secreted by macrophages and monocytes, increasing vascular permeability and endothelial activation and leading to blood–brain barrier breakdown. ICANS is not thought to be directly mediated by CAR-T cells themselves.

Risk factors for ICANS include high disease burden, older age, and the specific CAR-T product.

The onset of ICANS occurs (on average) approximately 5 days following CAR-T cell infusion and sometimes occurs concurrently with or shortly after cytokine release syndrome (CRS). However, in approximately 10% of patients, ICANS presents more than 3 weeks after CAR-T cell infusion.

Symptoms of ICANS are variable and can initially be vague. Patients experience mild tremor and confusion, which can then proceed to agitation, seizures, and cerebral oedema. A prominent and early feature of ICANS is hesitancy of speech and deterioration in handwriting, which can progress to aphasia with both expressive and receptive components, whereby the patient is alert but mute. The most devastating consequence of ICANS is the occurrence of status epilepticus, fatal cerebral oedema and occasionally intracerebral haemorrhage.

ICANS is a clinical diagnosis—brain MRI and CSF evaluation are rarely helpful but can be used to rule out alternative diagnoses, e.g., CNS infection. The EEG

J. H. Rees (✉)
National Hospital for Neurology and Neurosurgery, University College London Hospitals NHS Trust, London, UK

UCL Institute of Neurology, London, UK
e-mail: jeremy.rees@ucl.ac.uk

© The Author(s) 2022
N. Kröger et al. (eds.), *The EBMT/EHA CAR-T Cell Handbook*,
https://doi.org/10.1007/978-3-030-94353-0_27

Table 27.1 Immune Effector Cell Encephalopathy (ICE) Score

Immune Effector Cell Encephalopathy (ICE) Score
• *Orientation:* Orientation to year, month, city, hospital: 4 points
• *Naming:* Ability to name 3 objects (e.g., point to clock, pen, button): 3 points
• *Following commands:* Ability to follow simple commands (e.g., "show me 2 fingers" or "close your eyes and stick out your tongue"): 1 point
• *Writing:* Ability to write a standard sentence (e.g., "our national bird is the bald eagle"): 1 point
• *Attention:* Ability to count backwards from 100 by 10: 1 point

recording can be normal but can also demonstrate a pattern of variable abnormalities, including nonconvulsive status epilepticus.

Most cases spontaneously resolve, often with supportive care and early intervention with corticosteroid therapy.

All patients should be proactively monitored for ICANS twice daily to assess subtle changes in cognition using the 10-point Immune Effector Cell Encephalopathy (ICE) score (Table 27.1), which evaluates orientation, attention, writing, and language. This score is then integrated into an overall assessment of neurological function incorporating seizure activity, change in consciousness level, motor findings, and elevation in intracerebral pressure/cerebral oedema to obtain an ICANS grade. The higher the ICE score is, the lower the ICANS grade. Any patient with an ICE score less than 2 or with seizures is classified as severe (grade 3 or 4) and should be transferred to intensive care. Factors associated with a higher risk of ≥ grade 3 ICANS include a higher disease burden, low platelet count, and the development of early and severe CRS.

Management of ICANS is based on the severity of the score and the concurrence of CRS. Management is supportive for grade 1 ICANS, and dexamethasone with rapid taper is given for grade ≥2 ICANS. Suggested doses include 10–20 mg intravenous dexamethasone every 6 h for grades 2–3 and 1 g IV methylprednisolone for at least 3 days for grade 4 until symptoms improve. Seizures are treated with levetiracetam and status epilepticus with benzodiazepines. We do not recommend the use of prophylactic anti-epileptic drugs.

Other experimental approaches to the management of ICANS have been directed at controlling the potency of the CAR itself. Several CAR constructs have been designed with "suicide switches" or as "tunable CARs" by incorporating mechanisms designed to turn off or downgrade the CAR in the event of severe toxicity. In severe unresponsive cases, anakinra (IL-1 receptor antagonist) or chemotherapy to kill the CAR-T cells have been used. However, most cases resolve and do not result in residual neurocognitive damage (Tables 27.2 and 27.3).

Key Points
- ICANS is a common and usually reversible toxicity of CAR-T cell therapy, occurring within a week of infusion, often after cytokine release syndrome.
- ICANS is a clinical diagnosis—common early symptoms include word finding difficulties, confusion, and impaired fine motor skills. Investigations are rarely helpful except to rule out an alternative diagnosis, such as CNS infection.
- Severe ICANS consists of seizures, coma, and cerebral oedema and requires ITU care.
- Management of ICANS is largely supportive and depends on severity. Corticosteroids are the mainstay of care for all but Grade I ICANS and should be prescribed at high doses with a rapid taper.
- The prognosis is good, and the majority of patients fully recover without any long-term sequelae.

Table 27.2 American Society for Transplantation and Cellular Therapy (ASTCT) ICANS Consensus Grading for Adults

Overall ICANS Grade
Grade 1
Grade 2
Grade 3
Grade 4
ICE score[a]
7–9
3–6
0–2
0 (patient is unarousable and unable to perform the ICE assessment)
Depressed level of consciousness[b]
Awakens spontaneously
Awakens to voice
Awakens only to tactile stimulus
Patient is unarousable or requires vigorous or repetitive tactile stimuli to arouse. Stupor or coma
Seizure
N/A
N/A
Any clinical seizure focal or generalized that resolves rapidly or nonconvulsive seizures on EEG that resolve with intervention
Life-threatening prolonged seizure (>5 min) or repetitive clinical or electrical seizures without return to baseline in between

(continued)

Table 27.2 (continued)

Motor findings[c]
N/A
N/A
N/A
Deep focal motor weakness, such as hemiparesis or paraparesis

Elevated ICP/cerebral oedema
N/A
N/A
Focal/local oedema on neuroimaging[d]
Diffuse cerebral oedema on neuroimaging; decerebrate or decorticate posturing; Sixth nerve palsy; papilloedema; or Cushing's triad

ICANS grade is determined by the most severe event (ICE score, level of consciousness, seizure, motor findings, raised ICP/cerebral oedema) not attributable to any other cause; for example, a patient with an ICE score of 3 who has a generalized seizure is classified as having grade 3 ICANS

N/A indicates not applicable

[a]A patient with an ICE score of 0 may be classified as having grade 3 ICANS if awake with global aphasia, but a patient with an ICE score of 0 may be classified as having grade 4 ICANS if unarousable

[b] Depressed level of consciousness should be attributable to no other cause (e.g., no sedating medication)

[c] Tremors and myoclonus associated with immune effector cell therapies may be graded according to CTCAE v5.0, but they do not influence ICANS grading

[d] Intracranial haemorrhage with or without associated oedema is not considered a neurotoxicity feature and is excluded from ICANS grading. It may be graded according to CTCAE v5.0

Table 27.3 Approach to management of ICANS

ICANS Grade	Management
Grade 1	Consider levetiracetam seizure prophylaxis (750 mg BD)
	Avoid medications that cause central nervous system depression
	Seek neurology specialist consultation
	Supportive care
	Fundoscopic examination to assess for papilloedema
	Brain MRI with contrast (brain CT if brain MRI is not feasible)
	Consider diagnostic lumbar puncture with measurement of opening pressure where possible, sending samples for culture and sensitivity, cytology, biochemistry, and virology as a minimum
	Consider spine MRI if the patient has focal peripheral neurological deficits
	Consider electroencephalogram (EEG)
	Consider tocilizumab 8 mg/kg but only if concurrent CRS
	Twice daily neurocognitive assessment using the ICE score and ICANS grading
Grade 2	Investigations and supportive care as per grade 1
	Consider dexamethasone at a high dose with rapid weaning
	Consider transferring the patient to the intensive care unit (ICU)

Table 27.3   (continued)

ICANS Grade	Management
Grade 3	Investigations and supportive care as per grade 1 Administer dexamethasone 10–20 mg IV every 6 h or methylprednisolone equivalent until improvement to grade 1 and then taper Management of seizures with lorazepam 0.5 mg IV or other benzodiazepines as needed, followed by loading with levetiracetam or other anticonvulsants as required If fundoscopy reveals stage 1 or 2 papilloedema with cerebrospinal fluid (CSF) opening pressure > 20 mmHg, seek urgent advice from neurologist Consider repeat neuroimaging (CT or MRI) every 2–3 days if the patient has persistent grade ≥ 3 ICANS
Grade 4	Investigations and supportive care as per grade 1 Transfer patient to intensive care unit (ICU); consider mechanical ventilation for airway protection Seizure management as per grade 3 For convulsive status epilepticus, seek urgent advice from neurologist Administer methylprednisolone 1000 mg/day for 3 days, then taper at 250 mg every 12 hrs for 2 days, then 125 mg every 12 hrs for 2 days, then 60 mg every 12 hrs for 2 days For management of raised intracranial pressure, consider acetazolamide 1000 mg IV, followed by 250–1000 mg IV every 12 h; elevating the head of the bed; hyperventilation; and hyperosmolar therapy with mannitol

Further Reading

Neill L, Rees J, Roddie C. Neurotoxicity – CAR-T cell therapy: what the neurologist needs to know. Pract Neurol. 2020;20:287–95. https://doi.org/10.1136/practneurol-2020-002550.

Rubin DB, Danish HH, Ali AB, et al. Neurological toxicities associated with chimeric antigen receptor T-cell therapy. Brain. 2019;142:1334–48. https://doi.org/10.1093/brain/awz053.

Tallantyre EC, Evans NA, Parry-Jones J, et al. Neurological updates: neurological complications of CAR-T therapy. J Neurol. 2021;268:1544–54. https://doi.org/10.1007/s00415-020-10237-3.

Management of Hypogammaglobulinaemia and B-Cell Aplasia

28

Max Topp and Tobias Feuchtinger

The development and regulatory approval of CAR-T cell therapies targeting B-lineage surface antigens (Maude et al. 2018), such as CD19 or CD22, represents a major milestone in cancer immunotherapy. This treatment results in the depletion of malignant and normal B cells and is associated with hypogammaglobulinaemia. These on-target, off-tumour toxicities may result in an increased risk of infection. Careful long-term follow-up assessment of patients receiving CAR-T cell therapy is important. Management of these on-target, off-tumour effects should be well coordinated between treatment and referring centres if the patient returns to local providers following therapy. Aims of this toxicity management:

- Prophylaxis of acute and chronic infections.
- Treatment of infections.
- Prevention of organ damage due to silent and/or chronic infections (e.g., bronchiectasis).
- Best-possible quality of life.

Monitoring B-cell aplasia provides information on two aspects of treatment. First, B-cell aplasia is a sign of functional CAR persistence and often shows longer persistence than direct detection of the CAR-T cells themselves. Monitoring B-cell aplasia can guide decisions on the interval of monitoring of the malignant disease (e.g., imaging, MRD) and subsequent allogeneic HSCT in cases of CAR-T cell failure. Therefore, B-cell aplasia should be monitored together with remission

M. Topp
Medizinischen Klinik und Polklinik II, Universitätsklinikum Würzburg, Würzburg, Germany
e-mail: Topp_M@ukw.de

T. Feuchtinger (✉)
Department Pediatric Hematology, Oncology Hemostaseology and Stem Cell Transplantation, Dr von Hauner Children's Hospital, University Hospital, LMU, Munich, Germany
e-mail: Tobias.Feuchtinger@med.uni-muenchen.de

© The Author(s) 2022
N. Kröger et al. (eds.), *The EBMT/EHA CAR-T Cell Handbook*,
https://doi.org/10.1007/978-3-030-94353-0_28

status and CAR persistence. Second, B-cell aplasia is a helpful parameter to guide tapering or continuation of IgG substitution. The evidence level for the recommendation concerning monitoring B-cell aplasia is based on expert opinion and may vary in different patient age groups.

Because anti-CD19 and anti-CD22 CAR-T cells attack B-lineage precursors, long-term hypogammaglobulinaemia or agammaglobulinaemia are commonly seen in patients after CAR-T cell treatment. In paediatric centres, it has been the standard of care to perform immunoglobulin replacement following CAR-T cell therapy (Maude et al. 2014). However, there is no consensus regarding systematic IgG supplementation in adults with plasma-cell aplasia and hypogammaglobulinaemia after CAR-T cell therapy. Since persistent B-cell aplasia is associated with sinopulmonary infections, notably with encapsulated bacteria (Fishman et al. 2019), intravenous immunoglobulin replacement is performed in all patients with hypogammaglobulinaemia plus recurrent or chronic infections, especially pneumonia. After allogeneic HSCT plus CAR-T cell therapy, patients face an increased risk of infection-related morbidity and hence may require intensified (perhaps lifelong) IgG substitution regimens.

The duration of IgG substitution may be lifelong or last at least until recovery of functional B cells and plasma cells. However, data regarding the efficacy of prophylactic IgG replacement in CAR-T cell therapy recipients are limited (Hill et al. 2019), and current expert recommendations (Mahadeo et al. 2019, Yakoub-Agha et al. 2020) are extrapolated from the data for individuals with primary immune deficiencies (Perez et al. 2017, Picard et al. 2018). The long-term follow-up data from patients with Bruton agammaglobulinaemia provide a rationale to closely monitor immunoglobulin levels and acute, chronic and especially silent infections to prevent organ damage and maintain long-term quality of life. Individualized regimens aim to maintain serum immunoglobulin levels above 400 µg/l in adults and age-adapted normal ranges for children. Intravenous immunoglobulins (IVIGs) are usually given every 3–6 weeks or subcutaneously weekly (SCIGs). IVIG doses start at 0.4 g/kg body weight and SCIG doses at 0.1–0.15 g/kg body weight. Doses and intervals are adapted due to infections and serum IgG levels. After reaching a steady state, serum IgG levels should be controlled at least every 3 months.

Studies are needed to establish evidence-based approaches for management of B-cell aplasia and hypogammaglobulinaemia. Prophylactic immunoglobulin administration in this context and strategies may differ by patient and CAR-T cell product characteristics.

Key Points
- Long-term (potentially lifelong) monitoring of B-cell aplasia and IgG levels is necessary after CD19/CD22 targeting CAR-T cell therapies.
- Maintain serum immunoglobulin levels at physiologic levels through regular intravenous or subcutaneous substitution.
- The evidence level of this recommendation is at the expert opinion level.

References

Fishman JA, Hogan JI, Maus MV. Inflammatory and Infectious Syndromes Associated With Cancer Immunotherapies. Clin Infect Dis. 2019;69(6):909–20.

Hill JA, Giralt S, Torgerson TR, Lazarus HM. CAR-T - and a side order of IgG, to go? - Immunoglobulin replacement in patients receiving CAR-T cell therapy. Blood Rev. 2019;38:100596. e-pub ahead of print 2019/08/17

Mahadeo KM, Khazal SJ, Abdel-Azim H, Fitzgerald JC, Taraseviciute A, Bollard CM, et al. Management guidelines for paediatric patients receiving chimeric antigen receptor T cell therapy. Nat Rev Clin Oncol. 2019;16(1):45–63. e-pub ahead of print 2018/08/08

Maude SL, Frey N, Shaw PA, Aplenc R, Barrett DM, Bunin NJ, et al. Chimeric antigen receptor T cells for sustained remissions in leukemia. N Engl J Med. 2014;371(16):1507–17. e-pub ahead of print 2014/10/16

Maude SL, Laetsch TW, Buechner J, Rives S, Boyer M, Bittencourt H, et al. Tisagenlecleucel in children and young adults with B-cell lymphoblastic leukemia. N Engl J Med. 2018;378(5):439–48.

Perez EE, Orange JS, Bonilla F, Chinen J, Chinn IK, Dorsey M, et al. Update on the use of immunoglobulin in human disease: A review of evidence. J Allergy Clin Immunol. 2017;139(3S):S1–S46. e-pub ahead of print 2017/01/04

Picard C, Bobby Gaspar H, Al-Herz W, Bousfiha A, Casanova JL, Chatila T, et al. International Union of Immunological Societies: 2017 Primary immunodeficiency diseases committee report on inborn errors of immunity. J Clin Immunol. 2018;38(1):96–128. e-pub ahead of print 2017/12/12

Yakoub-Agha I, Chabannon C, Bader P, Basak GW, Bonig H, Ciceri F, et al. Management of adults and children undergoing chimeric antigen receptor T-cell therapy: best practice recommendations of the European Society for Blood and Marrow Transplantation (EBMT) and the Joint Accreditation Committee of ISCT and EBMT (JACIE). Haematologica. 2020;105(2):297–316. e-pub ahead of print 2019/11/23

Management of Myelotoxicity (Aplasia) and Infectious Complications

29

Marion Subklewe and Reuben Benjamin

Haematologic toxicity is the most common adverse event after CAR-T cell therapy, with a cumulative 1-year incidence of 58% (CTCAE grade $\geq$ 3) in the real-world setting (Wudhikarn et al., Blood Advances 2020). It is characterized by a biphasic temporal course and is often prolonged (Fried et al., Bone Marrow Transplant 2019, Rejeski et al., Blood et al. 2021a, b, Fig. 29.1). In a report of Axi-Cel-treated patients, only 30% demonstrated a neutrophil count $>1 \times 10^9$/L and 50% showed a platelet count $>50 \times 10^9$/L at 30 days following CAR-T cell treatment (Jain et al., Blood Advances 2020). In a long-term follow-up study of patients with ongoing CR and an absence of MDS, 16% of patients experienced prolonged significant cytopenias that lasted up to 22 months after CAR-T cell treatment (Cordeiro et al., Biol Blood Marrow Transplant 2020). These findings highlight that cytopenia can present long after lymphodepletion and the resolution of acute CRS. Risk factors include severe CRS/ICANS, cytopenia prior to initiation of lymphodepleting chemotherapy, and prior allogeneic stem cell transplantation (Jain et al., Blood Advances 2020, Fried et al., BMT, 2019). Importantly, cytopenia predisposes patients to severe infectious complications, which are the most frequent cause of non-relapse mortality (Nastoupil et al., JCO 2020).

The use of growth factors to manage early cytopenias after CAR-T cell therapy remains controversial. Cytokine profiles and mouse xenograft models have implicated GM-CSF in the pathogenesis of CRS and neuroinflammation (Sterner et al., Blood 2019). Accordingly, current recommendations discourage the use of GM-CSF and to initiate G-CSF only after resolution of CRS and/or ICANS (Yakoub-Agha et al., Haematologica 2020). However, in a report by Galli et al., prophylactic

M. Subklewe (✉)
Med. Klinik & Poliklinik III, LMU – Klinikum der Universität München, München, Germany
e-mail: Marion.Subklewe@med.uni-muenchen.de

R. Benjamin
King's College Hospital, London, UK
e-mail: reuben.benjamin@kcl.ac.uk

N. Kröger et al. (eds.), *The EBMT/EHA CAR-T Cell Handbook*,
https://doi.org/10.1007/978-3-030-94353-0_29

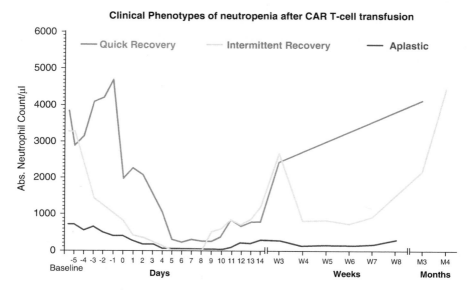

Fig. 29.1 Clinical Phenotypes of neutropenia (adapted from Rejeski et al., Blood 2021a, b)

G-CSF was used safely in 42 patients with grade 4 neutropenia on day 5 after CAR-T cell infusion, with no increased risk of CRS or ICANS and no negative impact on disease outcomes (Galli et al., Bone Marrow Transplantation 2020). Further studies are needed to identify patients at high risk for prolonged neutropenia and with an increased risk of infection that will benefit from early G-CSF initiation. The diagnostic workup for patients with prolonged cytopenia unresponsive to G-CSF should include screening for haematinic deficiency, viral infections (e.g., CMV, EBV, Hepatitis B/C, Parvovirus B19), concomitant myelosuppressive drugs (e.g., co-trimoxazole), secondary haemophagocytic lymphohistiocytosis, and the presence of disease in the bone marrow. In the event of severe bone marrow aplasia unresponsive to G-CSF, autologous or allogeneic stem cell rescue may be considered where possible (Rejeski et al., BMC ID 2021a, b, Godel et al., Haemasphere 2021). Other options include anti-inflammatory therapy (e.g., dexamethasone, anti-IL-6 blocking therapy) and thrombopoietin receptor agonists (e.g., eltrombopag) (Fig. 29.2).

Infections are another significant complication of CAR-T therapy as a result of prolonged neutropenia, long-term CD4 T cell lymphopenia, or B-cell aplasia (Hill and Seo et al., Blood 2020a, b). Other risk factors associated with infections include higher CRS grade and use of immunosuppressive agents, such as steroids, tocilizumab, and anakinra. The majority of infections occur early within the first 28 days, with bacterial infections being the most common, followed by viral and fungal infections. Late infections, especially with respiratory viruses, are also seen up to 90 days post CAR-T therapy (Cordeiro et al., BBMT 2020). Invasive fungal

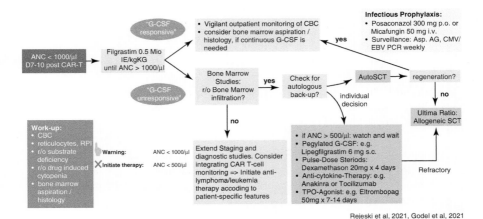

Rejeski et al, 2021, Godel et al, 2021
Hill and Seo et al, Blood Advances 2020

Fig. 29.2   Treatment algorithm for CD19 CAR-T cell-associated myelotoxicity

infections, both yeasts and moulds, have been reported in 1–15% of CAR-T-treated patients.

The use of antiviral, antifungal, and anti-pneumocystis (PCP) prophylaxis to reduce the risk of infections post-CAR-T cell therapy is recommended; however, there is no consensus on the optimal choice and duration of prophylaxis. Patients typically receive acyclovir or valacyclovir, yeast or mould-active antifungal prophylaxis, and co-trimoxazole to prevent PCP. Patients considered "high risk" for mould infections based on pre-infusion neutropenia, history of mould infection within 6 months, prior allo-SCT or underlying diagnosis of acute leukaemia as well as those who have had post-infusion grade ≥ 3 CRS/ICANS or prolonged treatment with steroids or other immunosuppressants should be offered mould-active prophylaxis. In the absence of high-risk factors, yeast-active prophylaxis may be sufficient, with pre-emptive monitoring for moulds recommended (Garner et al., J Fungi 2021). Antifungal prophylaxis is generally continued until recovery of the neutrophil count and cessation of immunosuppressants. PCP prophylaxis is typically given for 6 months or until the CD4 T cell count is >200 cells/μl. Monthly intravenous immunoglobulins may be considered when there is persistent severe hypogammaglobulinaemia and a history of recurrent infections. Treatment of suspected/confirmed infections post CAR-T therapy should follow Institutional guidelines and is generally similar to the management of infections after stem cell transplantation. The efficacy of vaccination following administration of CD19- or BCMA-targeted CAR-T cells remains unknown, but patients do need to be considered for vaccination at 6 months post-CAR-T therapy and guided by post-vaccine antibody titres (Hill et al., Blood 2020a, b). Effective strategies to prevent and manage infectious complications following CAR-T cell infusion are crucial in improving the outcomes of this promising therapy.

> **Key Points**
> - Haematological toxicity is the most common adverse event after CD19-specific CAR-T cell therapy and can predispose patients to severe infectious complications.
> - Administering prophylactic *G-CSF* from day 5 in neutropenic patients does not increase the incidence of severe CRS/ICANS and is safe in preserving CAR-T antilymphoma activity. Evidence level III-B.
> - Post-CART immunosuppression is multifactorial (e.g., neutropenia, lymphopenia, steroid use, B-cell aplasia, and hypogammaglobulinaemia), and infections significantly contribute to non-relapse mortality.
> - Anti-infective prophylaxis should follow institutional guidelines based on the patient-specific risk factors.

References

Cordeiro A, et al. Late events after treatment with CD19-targeted chimeric antigen receptor modified T cells. Biol Blood Marrow Transplant. 2020;26(1):26–33.

Fried S, et al. Early and late hematologic toxicity following CD19 CAR-T cells. Bone Marrow Transplant. 2019;54(10):1643–50.

Galli E, Allain V, Blasi R, Bernad S, Vercellino L, Morin F, Moatti H, Caillat-Zucman S, Chevret S, Thieblemont C. G-CSF does not worsen toxicities and efficacy of CAR-T cells in refractory/relapsed B-cell lymphoma. Bone Marrow Transplant. 2020;55:2347–9.

Goedel P, Sieg N, Heger JM, Kutsch N, Herling C, Bärmann B-N, Scheid C, Borchmann HU. Hematologic rescue of CAR-T cell mediated prolonged pancytopenia using autologous peripheral blood hematopoietic stem cells in a lymphoma patient. Hema. 2021;5(3):e545.

Hill JA, Seo SK. How I prevent infections in patients receiving CD19-targeted chimeric antigen receptor T cells for B-cell malignancies. Blood. 2020b;136(8):925–35.

Hill JH, Seo S. How I prevent infections in patients receiving CD19-targeted chimeric antigen receptor T cells for B-cell malignancies. Blood. 2020a;136(8):925–35.

Jain T, et al. Hematopoietic recovery in patients receiving chimeric antigen receptor T-cell therapy for hematologic malignancies. Blood Adv. 2020;4(15):3776–87.

Nastoupil LJ, Jain MD, Feng L, et al. Standard-of-care Axicabtagene Ciloleucel for relapsed or refractory large B-cell lymphoma: results from the US lymphoma CAR-T consortium. J Clin Oncol. 2020;38(27):3119–28.

Rejeski, K et al, *CAR-HEMATOTOX: A model for CAR-T cell related hematological toxicity in relapsed/refractory large B-cell lymphoma.* Blood 2021a Jun 24; online ahead of print.

Rejeski K, Kunz WG, Rudelius M, Bücklein V, Blumenerg V, Schmidt C, Karschnia P, Schöberl F, Dimitriadis K, Von Baumgarten L, Stemmler J, Weigert O, Dreyling M, Von Bergwelt-Baildon M, Subklewe M. Severe Candida glabrata pancolitis and fatal Aspergillus fumigatus pulmonary infection in the setting of bone marrow aplasia after CD19-directed CAR-T cell therapy- a case report. BMC Infect Dis. 2021b;21(1):121.

Sterner R, Sakemura R, Cox M, Yang N, Khadka R, Forsman C, Hansen M, Jin F, Ayssoufi K, Hefazi M, Schick K, Walters D, Chappell D, Ahmed O, Sahmoud t, Durrant C, Nevala W., Patnaik M, Pease L, Hedin K, Kay N, Johnson A, Kenderian S. CM-SF inhibition reduces CRS and neuroinflammation but enhances CAR-T cell function in xenografts. Blood. 2019;133(7):697–709.

Will Garner W, Samanta P, Haidar G. Invasive fungal infections after anti-CD19 chimeric antigen receptor-modified T-cell therapy: state of the evidence and future directions. J Fungi. 2021;7:156.

Wudhikarn K, et al. DLBCL patients treated with CD19 CAR-T cells experience a high burden of organ toxicities but low nonrelapse mortality. Blood Adv. 2020;4(13):3024–33.

Yakoub-Agha I, Chabannon C, Bader P, Basak GW, Bonig H, Ciceri F, Corbacioglu S, Duarte RF, Einsele H, Hudecek M, Kersten MJ, Köhl U, Kuball J, Mielke S, Mohty M, Murray J, Nagler A, Robinson S, Saccardi R, Sanchez-Guijo F, Snowden JA, Srour M, Styczynski J, Urbano-Ispizua A, Hayden PJ, Kröger N. Management of adults and children undergoing chimeric antigen receptor T-cell therapy: best practice recommendations of the European Society for Blood and Marrow Transplantation (EBMT) and the joint accreditation committee of ISCT and EBMT (JACIE). Haematologica. 2020;105(2):297–316.

Hermann Einsele ⓘ and Ibrahim Yakoub-Agha ⓘ

Secondary haemophagocytic lymphohistiocytosis (sHLH) or macrophage activation syndrome (MAS) is a life-threatening hyperinflammatory syndrome that can occur in patients with severe infections, e.g., COVID-19 infection, malignancy or autoimmune diseases. It is also a rare complication of allogeneic haematopoietic cell transplantation (allo-HCT), independent of the underlying trigger mechanism or underlying disorders associated with high mortality. There have been increasing reports of sHLH/MAS occurrence following CAR-T cell therapy, but its differentiation from cytokine release syndrome (CRS) is often difficult (Sandler et al. 2020).

The diagnosis of sHLH/MAS post-HCT requires observation of the clinical signs and symptoms of hyperinflammation, which can overlap with the symptoms of cytokine release syndrome or infectious complications, requiring a differential diagnosis. Typically, these symptoms include fever, cytopenia of more than one lineage, and multiorgan failure. Persistent fever without an identified infective cause or worsening fever in patients who have been treated for infection should prompt screening for sHLH/MAS (Karakike and Giamarellos-Bourboulis 2019). Serum ferritin is a suitable and readily available biomarker of sHLH/MAS and can also be used to monitor response to treatment.

CAR-T cell therapy, while emerging as an effective treatment for both haematological and nonhaematological malignancies, is associated with cytokine release syndrome (CRS), an acute toxicity resulting in hyperinflammation. Patients can present with CRS across a spectrum of severities, from low-grade constitutional symptoms to higher-grade systemic illness with multiorgan dysfunction, and in its

H. Einsele
Department of Internal Medicine II, University Hospital Würzburg, Würzburg, Bayern, Germany
e-mail: Einsele_h@ukw.de

I. Yakoub-Agha (✉)
Maladies du Sang, Unité de Thérapie Cellulaire, Centre hospitalier-Universitaire de Lille, Lille, France
e-mail: ibrahim.yakoubagha@chru-lille.fr

© The Author(s) 2022
N. Kröger et al. (eds.), *The EBMT/EHA CAR-T Cell Handbook*,
https://doi.org/10.1007/978-3-030-94353-0_30

most severe form, CRS can progress to fulminant sHLH/MAS. Neelapu et al. proposed diagnostic criteria for sHLH/MAS in patients with CRS post-CAR-T cell therapy demonstrating a peak serum ferritin measurement of >10,000 µg/L and two of the following findings: a grade > 3 increase in serum transaminase or bilirubin; grade > 3 oliguria or increase in serum creatinine; grade > 3 pulmonary oedema or histological evidence of haemophagocytosis in the bone marrow or organs (Neelapu et al. 2018) (Tables 30.1 and 30.2).

For effective treatment of sHLH/MAS, aggressive immunosuppression is required to control the hyperinflammatory state. Prompt recognition and treatment are important and reduce mortality. Corticosteroids remain the cornerstone of induction treatment, although over half of patients are steroid resistant (Fukaya et al. 2008) (Table 30.3).

Anakinra, an IL-1 antagonist, is effective in refractory sHLH/MAS and relatively safe in patients with sepsis (Shakoory et al. 2016) (Eloseily et al. 2019). Thus, anakinra has been used for refractory sHLH/MAS and was found to be effective in adult sHLH/MAS for patients with severe sHLH/MAS. Intravenous immunoglobulin (IVIG) infusions may also be effective in steroid-resistant and infection (EBV)-triggered sHLH/MAS (Chen et al. 1995).

A treatment protocol for sHLH/MAS accepting the heterogeneity of this syndrome has been recently published. The first-line treatment is intravenous

Table 30.1 Use of published criteria to support the diagnosis of sHLH/MAS after CAR-T cell therapy (adapted from Sandler et al. 2020)

Published criteria	Components of criteria	Centres (%)
HLH-2004 (for fHLH)	Molecular diagnosis consistent with HLH or 5/8 of the following: Fever, splenomegaly, bi or tri-lineage cytopenia, hypertriglyceridaemia ± hypofibrinogenaemia, haemophagocytosis on bone marrow biopsy, no diagnosis of malignancy, low/absent NK cell activity, raised ferritin, raised sIL-2r	43
H-score (for all SHLH/MAS)	Known underlying immunosuppression, fever, organomegaly, mono-, bi-, or tri-lineage Cytopenia, ferritin, triglycerides, fibrinogen, AST, haemophagocytosis on bone marrow biopsy. Overall score predicts likelihood of sHLH/MAS	16
Takagi et al. (for SHLH/MAS post-HSCT)	2 major or 1 major and all 4 minor criteria required. Major criteria: (A) engraftment delay, orumary or secondary failure or (B) histopathological evidence of haemophagocytosis. Minor criteria: fever, hepatosplenomegaly, elevated ferritin, elevated LDH.	10
PRINTO (for sHLH/MAS in sJIA)	Ferritin > 684µg/L and 2 of: platelets < 181 x 109, AST > 48 U/L, triglycerides > 256 mg/ dL, fibrinogen < 360 mg/ dL	1
MD Anderson (for sHLH/MAS post-CAR T cell therapy)	Ferritin of > 10,000 µg/L and 2 of: grade > 3 increase in serum transaminases or bilirubin: grade > 3 oliguria or increase in serum creatinine; grade > 3 pulmonary oedema; or histological evidence of haemophagocytosis in bone marrow or organs	7
Combination of the above		23

Table 30.2 The Hscore adapted to CAR-T cell therapy

Parameter	No. of points (criteria for scoring)
Temperature (°C)	0 (< 38,4), 33 (38,4-39,4), or 49 (> 39,4)
Organomegaly	0 (no), 23 (hepatomegaly or splenomegaly), or 38 (hepatomegaly and splenomegaly)
No. of cytopenias†	0 (1 lineage), 24 (2 lineages), or 34 (3 lineages)
Ferritin /ng/ml)	0 (<2,000), 35 (2,000-6,000), or 50 (>6,000)
Triglyceride (mmoles/liter)	0 (<1.5), 44 (1.5-4), or 64 (>4)
Fibrinogen (gm/liter)	0 (>2.5) or 30 (≤2.5)
Serum glutamic oxaloacetic transaminase (IU/liter)	0 (<30) or 19 (≥30)
Hemophagocytosis features on bone marrow aspirate	0 (no) or 35 (yes)

† Defined as a hemoglobin level of ≤9.2 gm/dl and/or a leukocyte count of ≤5,000/mm³ and/or a platelet count

Table 30.3   Use of published protocols in the management of sHLH/MAS post-HSCT or CAR-T cell therapy

Published protocol	Components of protocol	Centres (N)
MD Anderson (post CAR-T cell)	Supportive organ- specific treatment, broad-spectrum antibiotics, IV Tocilizumab or Siltuximab (anti-IL6 agents), IV corticosteroids	4
HLH-2004 (for fHLH)	8 weeks initial therapy with IV dexamethasone and Etoposide. Then ciclosporin is introduced, dexamethasone continues to be pulsed and etoposide continued whilst awaiting a donor for BMT	2
La Rosee et al.	Use of cortocosteroids +/- IVIG in most cases with addition of etoposide (if malignancy- triggered), ciclosporin & anakinra (if autoimmune- related) or anti-IL-6 (if CAR-T cell related)	1
HLH-94 (for fHLH)	8 weeks initial therapy with IV dexamethasone and Etoposide before proceeding to definitive treatment with BMT	1

methylprednisolone (IVMP) 1 g/day for 3–5 days plus IVIG 1 g/kg for 2 days, which can be repeated on day 14. If there is evidence of established sHLH/MAS or clinical deterioration, anakinra is added at 1–2 mg/kg daily, increasing up to 8 mg/kg/day. CSA is considered for early or steroid-resistant disease. Etoposide should be considered in refractory cases but can be problematic due to the already preexisting cytopenias in patients with sHLH/MAS following CAR-T cell therapy. Additionally, triggers, such as EBV, bacterial infection or underlying malignancy, particularly lymphoma, should be screened for and treated if adequately defined (Vatsayan et al. 2016).

Considerations for Patients Undergoing CAR-T Cell Therapy

- Steroids remain the cornerstone for sHLH/MAS treatment, but 50% of patients are resistant.
- A recent recommendation for HLH/MAS after CAR-T therapy:
  - Methylprednisolone 1 g/day for 3–5 days + IVIG 1 g/kg for 2 days, repeated on day 14.
  - In the case of deterioration, IV anakinra can be added up to 100 mg x 4/day.
  - Etoposide for refractory cases.
- Other treatments for sHLH/MAS after CAR-T cell therapy.
  - Ruxolitinib: found to be effective in a case report and small phase 1 study
- Cytokine blockers might be used
- IVIG: might be effective, especially if the underlying cause is infection.

Key Points
- Patients with persistent fever without an identified infection should be screened for sHLH/MAS.
- Serum ferritin is a suitable and readily available biomarker of sHLH/MAS.
- Corticosteroids are the cornerstone of induction treatment.
- >50% of patients are steroid-refractory.
- IV anakinra is the second line treatment.
- Etoposide can be used in refractory sHLH/MAS.

References

Chen RL, Lin KH, Lin DT, Su IJ, Huang LM, Lee PI, et al. Immunomodulation treatment for childhood virus-associated haemophagocytic lymphohistiocytosis. Br J Haematol. 1995;89:282–90.

Eloseily EM, Weiser P, Crayne CB, Haines H, Mannion ML, Stoll ML, et al. Benefit of anakinra in treating pediatric secondary hemophagocytic lymphohistiocytosis. Arthritis Rheumatol. 2019;72:326–34.

Fukaya S, Yasuda S, Hashimoto T, Oku K, Kataoka H, Horita T, et al. Clinical features of Haemophagocytic syndrome in patients with systemic autoimmune diseases: analysis of 30 cases. Rheumatology. 2008;47:1686–91.

Karakike E, Giamarellos-Bourboulis EJ. Macrophage activation-like syndrome: a distinct entity leading to early death in sepsis. Front Immunol. 2019;10:55.

Neelapu SS, Tummala S, Kebriaei P, Wierda W, Gutierrez C, Locke FL, et al. Chimeric antigen receptor T-cell therapy – assessment and management of toxicities. Nat Rev Clin Oncol. 2018;15:47–62.

Sandler RD, Tattersall RS, Schoemans H, Greco R, Badoglio M, Labopin M, Alexander T, Kirgizov K, Rovira M, Saif M, Saccardi R, Delgado J, Peric Z, Koenecke C, Penack O, Basak G, Snowden JA. Diagnosis and Management of Secondary HLH/MAS Following HSCT and CAR-T Cell Therapy in Adults; A Review of the Literature and a Survey of Practice Within EBMT Centres on Behalf of the Autoimmune Diseases Working Party (ADWP) and Transplant Complications Working Party (TCWP). Front Immunol. 2020;31(11):524.

Shakoory B, Carcillo JA, Chatham WW, Amdur RL, Zhao H, Dinarello CA, et al. Interleukin-1 receptor blockade is associated with reduced mortality in sepsis patients with features of macrophage activation syndrome: reanalysis of a prior phase III trial. Critical Care Med. 2016;44:275–81.

Vatsayan A, Cabral L, Abu-Arja R. Hemophagocytic lymphohistiocytosis (HLH) after hematopoietic stem cell transplant (HSCT) or an impostor: a word of caution! Blood Marrow Transplant. 2016;22:S262–3.

ICU

31

Udo Holtick and Elie Azoulay

CAR-T cell treatment comes with significant side effects that challenge the structure and capacity of haematology wards and will regularly necessitate intermittent patient transfer to the ICU. Life-threatening adverse events include cytokine release syndrome and immune effector cell-associated neurotoxicity syndrome, which can occur within hours or days after administration. Sepsis might also require ICU admission within the days that follow CAR-T infusion in these high-risk immunocompromised patients.

Critical care and ICU specialists play an important role in the management of patients receiving CAR-T therapies. A substantial number of patients require an ICU bed, and CRS is the leading reason for ICU admission (Fitzgerald et al. 2017; Gutierrez et al. 2020). Prompt and appropriate ICU management relies on a fine-tuned dialogue between haematologists and ICU specialists and on an appropriate definition of the threshold moment to target ICU admission. Hence, less than half of patients require high-dose vasopressors, mechanical ventilation, or renal replacement therapy (Azoulay et al. 2020). However, critical care also benefits those in whom appropriate antibiotics, source control of sepsis, echo-guided fluid expansion, prevention of acute kidney injury, and an optimal oxygenation strategy are provided.

In some patients with comorbidities, the role of ICU specialists starts at the time of patient eligibility for CAR-T cell therapy. Evaluation of patient frailty and risk for developing organ dysfunction and sepsis helps define the optimal timing of ICU admission. When patients are starting lymphodepletion, the ICU specialists at least receive a transmission. Of course, when patients have persistent stage 1 or stage 2

U. Holtick (✉)
Department I of Internal Medicine, University Hospital Cologne, Cologne, Germany
e-mail: Udo.holtick@uk-koeln.de

E. Azoulay
Critical Care Department, Saint-Louis Hospital, Paris University, Paris, France
e-mail: Elie.azoulay@aphp.fr

© The Author(s) 2022
N. Kröger et al. (eds.), *The EBMT/EHA CAR-T Cell Handbook*,
https://doi.org/10.1007/978-3-030-94353-0_31

CRS, again, the ICU specialist is alerted. Overall, these careful strategies have allowed a reduction in the need for ICU admission, with the numbers balanced with widespread use of cell therapy and immunotherapy worldwide, which has been helpful in a setting of scarce ICU beds.

To optimally manage CAR-T recipients, haematologists, oncologists, and intensivists need to acquire the necessary knowledge and skills. Transdisciplinary meetings ease harmonization of patient management, keeping all participants aware of the advances in each specialty. Until recently, the ICU has primarily been used as a bridge to cure patients with cancer (Azoulay et al. 2017; Gray et al. 2021). However, CAR-T cell therapy challenges these concepts, producing a time-limited trial that is offered to every CAR-T cell recipient, despite the underlying refractory malignancy, and significant hopes are put towards complete remission or bridging to another promising therapy. However, not all patients respond to treatment with CAR-T cells, and many patients ultimately relapse. Thus, we will need to adapt the approach to admission and discharge from the ICU in a context of uncertainty and with hope for recovery.

The key points below emphasize the role of the ICU specialist throughout the CAR-T cell recipient journey and proposes the importance of maintaining tight collaboration across the involved specialties.

Key Points

CAR-T cell therapy: Framework to emphasize multidisciplinary collaboration.

Adapted from Azoulay E et al., Am J Respir Crit Care Med. 2019

- Consultation with an ICU specialist to assess eligibility for CAR-T cell therapy and anticipate post-infusion risks; consultation at the time of lymphodepletion and once any sign of toxicity or sepsis occurs.
- Apply a common information network to share important information.
- Reach agreement on the goals of care.
- Time-limited trials should be considered for all CAR-T cell recipients.
- CRS and ICANS must be assessed clinically several times per day for at least 7 days.
- Elicit prompt ICU admission once CRS reaches grade II.
- Leverage the latest advances.
- Liaise with all stakeholders to facilitate research.
- Share experiences with other specialists.

References

Azoulay E, Darmon M, Valade S. Acute life-threatening toxicity from CAR-T cell therapy. Intensive Care Med. 2020;46(9):1723–6. https://doi.org/10.1007/s00134-020-06193-1.

Azoulay E, Schellongowski P, Darmon M, et al. The intensive care medicine research agenda on critically ill oncology and hematology patients. Intensive Care Med. 2017;19 https://doi.org/10.1007/s00134-017-4884-z.

Azoulay E, Shimabukuro-Vornhagen A, Darmon M, von Bergwelt-Baildon M. Critical Care Management of Chimeric Antigen Receptor T Cell-related Toxicity. Be aware and prepared. Am J Respir Crit Care Med. 2019;200(1):20–3. https://doi.org/10.1164/rccm.201810-1945ED.

Fitzgerald JC, Weiss SL, Maude SL, et al. Cytokine release syndrome after chimeric antigen receptor T cell therapy for acute lymphoblastic leukemia. Crit Care Med. 2017;45(2):e124–31. https://doi.org/10.1097/CCM.0000000000002053.

Gray TF, Temel JS, El-Jawahri A. Illness and prognostic understanding in patients with hematologic malignancies. Blood Rev. 2021;45:100692. https://doi.org/10.1016/j.blre.2020.100692.

Gutierrez C, Brown ART, Herr MM, et al. The chimeric antigen receptor-intensive care unit (CAR-ICU) initiative: surveying intensive care unit practices in the management of CAR-T cell associated toxicities. J Crit Care. 2020;58:58–64. https://doi.org/10.1016/j.jcrc.2020.04.008.

Post-CAR-T Cell Therapy (Consolidation and Relapse): Acute Lymphoblastic Leukaemia

32

Jordan Gauthier

Role of consolidative allogeneic haematopoietic cell transplantation (allo-HCT) for B-cell acute lymphoblastic leukaemia (B-ALL) patients in minimal residual disease-negative (MRD) complete remission (CR) after CD19 CAR-T cell therapy.

The role of consolidative allo-HCT in B-ALL patients achieving MRD-negative CR after CD19 CAR-T cell therapy is still debated. At the last update of the ELIANA clinical trial, which investigated tisagenlecleucel in children and young adults with relapsed or refractory (R/R) B-ALL, the median duration of remission and overall survival was not reached (median follow-up, 24 months). The 24-month relapse-free survival probability in responders was 62%, with plateauing of the probability curves after 1 year (Grupp et al. 2019). Consolidation with allo-HCT was reported in only 9% of CR patients, suggesting that CD19 CAR-T cell therapy alone with tisagenlecleucel may be curative in a significant proportion of paediatric patients. In contrast, to date, the data do not suggest that CD19 CAR-T cell therapy is a definitive approach in most adults with R/R B-ALL. Across the main academic and industry-sponsored clinical trials of CD19 CAR-T cell therapy for adult B-ALL, the median durations of response ranged from 8 to 19 months, with important variations in the proportion of patients receiving consolidative allo-HCT in CR after treatment (35–75%) (Shah et al. 2019; Frey et al. 2020; Hay et al. 2019; Park et al. 2018). In our experience, we observed favourable outcomes in patients undergoing allo-HCT while in MRD-negative CR after defined-composition CD19 CAR-T cell therapy, with 2-year EFS and OS probabilities of 61% and 72%, respectively. After adjusting for previously identified prognostic factors for event-free survival (EFS; pre-lymphodepletion LDH concentration and platelet count, cyclophosphamide-fludarabine lymphodepletion), the hazard ratio for allo-HCT was 0.39 (95% CI

J. Gauthier (✉)
Clinical Research Division, Fred Hutchinson Cancer Research Center, Seattle, WA, USA

Division of Medical Oncology, University of Washington, Seattle, WA, USA
e-mail: jgauthier@fredhutch.org

N. Kröger et al. (eds.), *The EBMT/EHA CAR-T Cell Handbook*,
https://doi.org/10.1007/978-3-030-94353-0_32

0.13–1.15, $p = 0.09$), suggesting a beneficial effect on EFS. Based on these findings, our approach in adult patients is to recommend consolidative allo-HCT in adult patients with R/R B-ALL in MRD-negative CR after CD19 CAR-T cell therapy. Additionally, patient age and preferences, comorbidities, a history of prior transplant, and MRD must be taken into account. Investigators from the NCI/NIH (Lee et al. 2016) and Seattle Children's Hospital (Summers et al. 2018) reported a survival advantage in children and young adults consolidated with allo-HCT after CD19 CAR-T cell therapy. However, notably, to date, the available data rely on nonrandomized, retrospective analyses, and are potentially subject to important biases (Suissa 2007; Lévesque et al. 2010).

Management of Relapsed B-ALL After CD19 CAR-T Cell Therapy

CD19-Positive Disease After CD19 CAR-T Cell Therapy

If cryopreserved end-manufacturing CAR-T cells are available and the target antigen is still expressed, an attractive approach is to use the "left-over" cells to manufacture a second CAR-T cell product. We have shown that second CD19 CAR-T cell infusions are feasible and well tolerated, but in most cases directed at the murine single chain variable fragment (scFv) CAR domain, antitumour efficacy is limited by anti-CAR immune responses. We observed superior outcomes in patients who received cyclophosphamide and fludarabine lymphodepletion prior to the first CAR-T cell infusion and who received a higher CAR-T cell dose (10 times higher than the first CAR-T cell infusion). However, second CAR-T cell infusions achieved a CR in only 3 of 14 ALL patients (21%) (Gauthier et al. 2020). Efforts are underway to mitigate or circumvent anti-CAR immune responses using a CAR comprising humanized or fully human scFvs (Gauthier et al. 2018; Brudno et al. 2020). Maude et al. evaluated the use of the humanized scFv-bearing CD19 CAR-T cell product CTL119 in 38 children and young adults (Grupp et al. 2015). MRD-negative CR could be achieved in murine CAR-exposed patients (43%), although at a lower rate than in the CAR-naïve population (100%). The 12-month relapse-free survival probabilities in responding patients were 82% and 56% in the CAR-exposed and CAR-naïve cohorts, respectively. In another report, Cao et al. observed CR in 2 of 5 patients previously exposed to murine CD19 CAR-T cells(Cao et al. 2019). Further studies are needed to determine whether immunogenicity, poor CAR-T cell function or disease-related factors underlie the reduced efficacy of CD19 CAR-T cells employing fully human or humanized scFv in the murine CAR-exposed setting.

CD19-Negative Disease After CD19 CAR-T Cell Therapy

Encouraging results have been reported using CD22-targeted CAR-T cells, including in patients with CD19-negative B-ALL blasts after prior CD19 CAR-T cell therapy. Shah et al. reported their experience in 58 children and young adults with

R/R B-ALL, including 62% of patients who were previously treated with a CD19 CAR-T cell product (Shah et al. 2020). CD22 CAR-T cells achieved an MRD-negative CR in 61% of cases, with a median duration of response of 6 months (13 of 35 MRD-negative CR patients [37%] went on to receive allo-HCT). The MRD-negative CR rate in patients previously treated with CD19 CAR-T cells was 64%. In another report from Pan et al., CD22 CAR-T cells were administered to 34 children and adult patients. Prior failure of CD19 CAR-T cell therapy was documented in 91% of patients. CD22 CAR-T cells achieved MRD-negative CRs in 76% of patients. Responses were durable, with a 1-year leukaemia-free survival probability of 58% in CR patients (11 of 30 CR patients [37%] went on to receive allo-HCT) (Pan et al. 2019).

Key Points
- When feasible, allo-HCT should be offered to adult patients with R/R B-ALL in MRD-negative CR after CD19 CAR-T cell therapy.
- CD22 CAR-T cells are associated with high response rates after CD19 CAR-T cell failure, and the most durable responses are observed after consolidative allo-HCT.
- CD19 CAR-T cells with fully human or humanized scFv are under investigation to mitigate anti-CAR immune responses, potentially impeding the efficacy of repeat CAR-T cell infusions.

References

Brudno JN, Lam N, Vanasse D, Shen YW, Rose JJ, Rossi J, et al. Safety and feasibility of anti-CD19 CAR-T cells with fully human binding domains in patients with B-cell lymphoma. Nat Med. 2020;26(2):270–80.

Cao J, Cheng H, Qi K, Chen W, Shi M, Zheng J, et al. Humanized CD19-specific chimeric antigen receptor T cells for acute lymphoblastic leukemia. Blood. 2019;134(Supplement_1):3872.

Frey NV, Shaw PA, Hexner EO, Pequignot E, Gill S, Luger SM, et al. Optimizing chimeric antigen receptor T-cell therapy for adults with acute lymphoblastic leukemia. J Clin Oncol. 2020;38(5):415–22.

Gauthier J, Bezerra E, Hirayama AV, Pender BS, Vakil A, Steinmetz RN, et al. Repeat infusions of CD19 CAR-T cells: factors associated with response, CAR-T cell in vivo expansion, and progression-free survival. ASTCT. 2020;26(3):S267–S8.

Gauthier J, Hirayama AV, Hay KA, Sheih A, Pender BS, Hawkins RM, et al. Immunotherapy with T-cells engineered with a chimeric antigen receptor bearing a human CD19-binding single chain variable fragment for relapsed or refractory acute lymphoblastic leukemia and B-cell non-Hodgkin lymphoma. Blood. 2018;132(Supplement 1):1415.

Grupp SA, Maude SL, Rives S, Baruchel A, Boyer M, Bittencourt H, et al. Tisagenlecleucel for the treatment of pediatric and young adult patients with relapsed/refractory acute lymphoblastic leukemia: updated analysis of the ELIANA clinical trial. Biol Blood Marrow Tr. 2019;25(3):S126–S7.

Grupp SA, Maude SL, Shaw PA, Aplenc R, Barrett DM. Durable remissions in children with relapsed/refractory ALL treated with T cells engineered with a CD19-targeted chimeric antigen receptor (CTL019). Blood. 2015;126(23):681.

Hay KA, Gauthier J, Hirayama AV, Voutsinas JM, Wu Q, Li D, et al. Factors associated with durable EFS in adult B-cell ALL patients achieving MRD-negative CR after CD19 CAR-T cell therapy. Blood. 2019;133(15):1652–63.

Lee DW, Stetler-Stevenson M, Yuan CM, Shah NN, Delbrook C, Yates B, et al. Long-term outcomes following CD19 CAR-T cell therapy for B-ALL are superior in patients receiving a Fludarabine/cyclophosphamide preparative regimen and post-CAR hematopoietic stem cell transplantation. Blood. 2016;128(22):218.

Lévesque LE, Hanley JA, Kezouh A, Suissa S. Problem of immortal time bias in cohort studies: example using statins for preventing progression of diabetes. BMJ. 2010;340(mar12 1):b5087.

Pan J, Niu Q, Deng B, Liu S, Wu T, Gao Z, et al. CD22 CAR-T cell therapy in refractory or relapsed B acute lymphoblastic leukemia. Leukemia. 2019;33(12):2854–66.

Park JH, Riviere I, Gonen M, Wang X, Senechal B, Curran KJ, et al. Long-term follow-up of CD19 CAR-therapy in acute lymphoblastic leukemia. N Engl J Med. 2018;378(5):449–59.

Shah BD, Bishop M, Oluwole OO, Logan A, Baer MR, Donnellan W, et al. End of phase I results of ZUMA-3, a phase 1/2 study of KTE-X19, anti-CD19 chimeric antigen receptor (CAR) T cell therapy, in adult patients (pts) with relapsed/refractory (R/R) acute lymphoblastic leukemia (ALL). ASCO. 2019;37(15_suppl):7006.

Shah NN, Highfill SL, Shalabi H, Yates B, Jin J, Wolters PL, et al. CD4/CD8 T-cell selection affects chimeric antigen receptor (CAR) T-cell potency and toxicity: updated results from a phase I anti-CD22 CAR-T cell trial. J Clin Oncol. 2020;38(17):1938–50.

Suissa S. Immortal time bias in observational studies of drug effects. Pharmacoepidem Dr S. 2007;16(3):241–9.

Summers C, Annesley C, Bleakley M, Dahlberg A, Jensen MC, Gardner R. Long term follow-up after SCRI-CAR19v1 reveals late recurrences as well as a survival advantage to consolidation with HCT after CAR-T cell induced remission. Blood. 2018;132(Supplement 1):967.

Post-CAR-T Cell Therapy (Consolidation and Relapse): Lymphoma

33

Didier Blaise and Sabine Fürst

Even after a decade of use, CAR-T cell therapy for non-Hodgkin lymphoma (NHL) is still evolving, and disease control is now the main concern in the majority of experienced centres. Indeed, despite highly appealing objective response (OR) rates in refractory patients, the long-term overall survival (OS) of this population has only slightly improved. Pivotal studies have suggested that 2-year OS rates do not surpass 30%, even though results improve when complete response (CR) is achieved within the first 3 months after treatment (Wang et al. 2020; Schuster et al. 2019; Neelapu et al. 2017). Although achieving this exceptionally high level of OR is praiseworthy, similar improvements have not been made regarding OS, and current OS probabilities are not satisfactory. Of course, there are multiple reasons for this; a substantial proportion of patients either do not achieve an initial response or experience progression very soon after treatment, with poor OS (Chow et al. 2019). Both populations present with disease burden or aggressive cancer prior to CAR-T cell therapy, possibly having been referred too late in the course of treatment or waited too long before CAR-T cells were processed for them. Both of these issues have potential solutions, such as more widely publicizing the efficacy of CAR-T cells, which may increase referrals at an earlier stage, and developing methods, which are already being heavily investigated, for shortening the manufacturing process (Rafiq et al. 2020). In the latter case, the use of allogeneic lymphocytes could allow for already prepared cells to be readily used when needed and would most likely be the most efficient strategy as long as the risk of graft-versus host disease is offset (Graham and Jozwik 2018). Thus, achieving CR is a crucial step in increasing OS, as patients with partial response (PR) or stable disease (SD) present with lower OS, while currently, recurrence appears to be rare when CR is maintained for more than 6 months (Komanduri 2021). However, the disease will likely recur in more than

D. Blaise (✉) · S. Fürst
Transplant and Cellular Immunotherapy Program, Department of Hematology, Institute Paoli-Calmettes, Marseille, France
e-mail: blaised@ipc.unicancer.fr; fursts@ipc.unicancer.fr

© The Author(s) 2022
N. Kröger et al. (eds.), *The EBMT/EHA CAR-T Cell Handbook*,
https://doi.org/10.1007/978-3-030-94353-0_33

half of patients in the months following treatment, possibly due to issues such as the poor persistence of CAR-T cells (which may not be as crucial as once thought for acute lymphoblastic leukaemia (Komanduri 2021)) or the loss of target antigen expression (which has been regularly documented (Rafiq et al. 2020)). Both of these mechanisms could potentially be used to develop methods that reduce recurrence after CAR-T cell therapy. In fact, the most popular approaches currently being investigated are attempting to either use two CAR-T cell types that each target different antigens or to create CAR-T cell constructs that target either multiple antigens or an antigen other than CD19 (Shah et al. 2020). The concomitant infusion of CAR-T cells with targeted therapies is also being explored in other B-cell malignancies and appears to both increase the CR rate and decrease recurrence (Gauthier et al. 2020). When recurrence does occur, patient OS is rather dismal, and the best remaining option would most likely be inclusion in a clinical trial. If this option is not available, salvage therapy may be attempted, although cytotoxic treatments are extremely limited given that most diseases have been refractory to numerous lines of treatment prior to immunotherapy. A few case reports and studies with a small patient population receiving anti-PD-1 antibodies, ibrutinib, or ImiDs have been reported with largely anecdotal supporting evidence (Byrne et al. 2019). However, even in the case of a new objective response (OR), the subsequent risk of recurrence is substantial and may invite further consolidation with allogeneic haematopoietic stem cell transplantation (Byrne et al. 2019), which has already been performed in patients treated for acute lymphoblastic leukaemia (Hay et al. 2019). However, the efficacy of this strategy remains to be validated in NHL patients in clinical trials. Further supporting evidence, although limited, has recently been reported concerning an additional treatment with CAR-T cells inducing an OR. Of the 21 NHL patients included in the study, the OR rate after the second infusion was 52% (CR, $n = 4$; PR, $n = 7$), with some durable responses inviting further investigations (Gauthier et al. 2021). Overall, with such poor outcomes after recurrence, current efforts are also focused on predicting the patients most likely to experience disease progression and that are potential candidates for preemptive consolidation therapy, although there is no doubt that patients who do not achieve a rapid CR should be the first candidates. Additionally, immune monitoring should encompass not only CAR-T cell survival but also the detection of circulating tumour DNA (Komanduri 2021) because this could aid in detecting subclinical recurrence and in deciding whether consolidation or maintenance therapy should be administered. However, currently, all these approaches are highly speculative and require further clinical study.

Key Points
- Relapse after CAR-T cell treatment for NHL is associated with a dismal outcome.
- Presently, there is no consensus on salvage therapy.
- Investigating methods to prevent recurrence is mandatory.
- Inclusion in clinical trials is recommended.

References

Byrne M, Oluwole OO, Savani B, et al. Understanding and managing large B cell lymphoma relapses after chimeric antigen receptor T cell therapy. Biol Blood Marrow Transplant. 2019;25(11):e344–51.

Chow VA, Gopal AK, Maloney DG, et al. Outcomes of patients with large B-cell lymphomas and progressive disease following CD19-specific CAR-T cell therapy. Am J Hematol. 2019;94(8):E209–13.

Gauthier J, Hirayama AV, Purushe J, et al. Feasibility and efficacy of CD19-targeted CAR-T cells with concurrent ibrutinib for CLL after ibrutinib failure. Blood. 2020;135(19):1650–60.

Gauthier J, Bezerra ED, Hirayama AV, et al. Factors associated with outcomes after a second CD19-targeted CAR-T cell infusion for refractory B-cell malignancies. Blood. 2021;137(3):323–35.

Graham C, Jozwik A. Pepper a et al allogeneic CAR-T cells: more than ease of access? Cell. 2018;7(10):5.

Hay KA, Gauthier J, Hirayama AV, et al. Factors associated with durable EFS in adult B-cell ALL patients achieving MRD-negative CR after CD19 CAR-T cell therapy. Blood. 2019;133(15):1652–63.

Komanduri KV. Chimeric antigen receptor T-cell therapy in the management of relapsed non-Hodgkin lymphoma. J Clin Oncol. 2021;39(5):476–86.

Neelapu SS, Locke FL, Bartlett NL, et al. Axicabtagene ciloleucel CAR-T cell therapy in refractory large B-cell lymphoma. N Engl J Med. 2017;377(26):2531–44.

Rafiq S, Hackett CS, Brentjens RJ. Engineering strategies to overcome the current roadblocks in CAR-T cell therapy. Nat Rev Clin Oncol. 2020;17(3):147–67.

Schuster SJ, Bishop MR, Tam CS, et al. Tisagenlecleucel in adult relapsed or refractory diffuse large B-cell lymphoma. N Engl J Med. 2019;380(1):45–56.

Shah NN, Johnson BD, Schneider D, et al. Bispecific anti-CD20, anti-CD19 CAR-T cells for relapsed B cell malignancies: a phase 1 dose escalation and expansion trial. Nat Med. 2020;26(10):1569–75.

Wang M, Munoz J, Goy A, et al. KTE-X19 CAR-T cell therapy in relapsed or refractory mantle-cell lymphoma. N Engl J Med. 2020;382(14):1331–42.

Post-CAR-T Cell Therapy (Consolidation and Relapse): Multiple Myeloma

34

Paula Rodríguez-Otero and Jesús F. San Miguel

Adoptive cell therapy with BCMA-directed autologous CAR-T cells has shown very encouraging results in end-stage relapse and refractory multiple myeloma (MM), with overall response rates ranging between 73% and 96.9%, complete response (CR) rates between 33% and 67.9%, and MRD negativity in 50–74% of patients in the two largest phase 2 studies of ide-cel (idecabtagene autoleucel, KarMMa) and cilta-cel (ciltacabtagene autoleucel, CARTITUDE 1) reported thus far (Madduri et al. 2020; Munshi et al. 2021). Unfortunately, responses are usually not maintained, and no plateau has yet been seen in the survival curves. The median progression-free survival (PFS) in the KarMMa study of ide-cel was 8.8 months (95% CI, 5.6–11.6) among all 128 patients infused, increased to 12.1 months (95% CI, 8.8–12.3) among patients receiving the highest dose (450×10^6 CAR + T cells) and increased to 20.2 months (95% CI, 12.3–NE) among those achieving a CR. In the CARTITUDE-1 study, with a median follow-up of 12.4 months, the median PFS has not yet been reached, and the 12-month PFS rate was 76.6% (95% CI; 66.0–84.3). The absence of a clear plateau in PFS differs from what has been observed in DLBCL or B-ALL with currently approved CD-19-directed CAR-T cells, where (albeit with a shorter PFS and lower rates of CR) patients remaining free from relapse beyond 6 months are likely to enjoy prolonged disease control or even be cured.

Mechanisms of resistance and relapse following CAR-T cell therapy in MM are poorly understood, and several factors may explain these differences in survival (D'Agostino and Raje 2020; Rodríguez-Otero et al. 2020). MM is a very heterogeneous disease with important clonal heterogeneity and a highly deregulated marrow microenvironment. In addition, CAR-T cell therapy has been evaluated in very heavily pretreated populations, with a significant proportion of patients being

P. Rodríguez-Otero · J. F. San Miguel (✉)
Department of Hematology, Clínica Universidad de Navarra, University of Navarra, Pamplona, Spain
e-mail: paurodriguez@unav.es; sanmiguel@unav.es

triple-class refractory and exposed to all available therapies, reflecting a difficult-to-treat population with an expected PFS of less than 4 months (Gandhi et al. 2019).

To maintain responses and prolong survival, different strategies are being investigated, such as dual targeting to prevent antigen loss (Jiang et al. 2020) and manufacturing changes to increase the proportion of long-lived T cells with a memory phenotype in the infused product, which has been associated with improved outcomes and longer CAR-T cell persistence (Alsina et al. 2020; Costello et al. 2019; Fraietta et al. 2018). The most advanced strategy to consolidate responses is combination with immunostimulatory drugs, such as IMIDs or checkpoint inhibitors, to improve functional CAR-T cell persistence and avoid exhaustion. Several clinical trials using these strategies are ongoing.

Interestingly, considering relapse after CAR-T cell therapy, emerging data show a discordance between PFS and overall survival (OS). In the updated results from the CRB-401 phase 1 study, the median PFS and OS reported were 8.8 (95% CI 5.9–11.9) and 34.2 (95% CI, 19.2–NE) months, respectively, across all doses (Lin et al. 2020). OS data in the KarMMa study are still immature, with 66% of patients censored overall (Munshi et al. 2021). Thus far, this gap between PFS and OS is not as clear in other studies, but the follow-up time is still very short for the majority of the trials. In the Legend-2 study, one of the BCMA studies with a longer follow-up time, the median PFS for all treated patients was 20 months, and the median OS was not reached, with an 18-month OS rate of 68% (Chen et al. 2019). This suggests that MM patients relapsing after CAR-T cell therapy may subsequently respond to salvage treatments, including drug combinations that have previously failed. One can speculate about potential modifications of the immune system or the bone marrow microenvironment induced by CAR-T cells. Unfortunately, data addressing this phenomenon are not yet available. Furthermore, CAR-T cell therapy has been shown to significantly improve health-related quality of life (Cohen et al. 2020; Martin III et al. 2020; Shah et al. 2020), and this better physical condition together with a prolonged treatment-free interval are two key factors that may predispose patients to accept additional rescue therapies, which would also contribute to the OS gain.

Unfortunately, data are not yet available to elucidate what optimal rescue therapies should be proposed after CAR-T cell progression. Anecdotal cases of patients progressing after BCMA-directed CAR-T cell infusion and then treated with other BCMA agents, such as belantamab mafodotin or checkpoint inhibitors, have been reported and showed that this approach has limited efficacy (Cohen et al. 2019). Nevertheless, the optimal approach in patients failing BCMA-directed CAR-T cell therapy will be to employ therapies with different mechanisms of action (Melflufen, CELMODs, Selinexor) or immunotherapies directed against different targets, such as SLAMF7, GPRC5D or FcRH5, using either bispecific T-cell engagers (Talquetamab or Cevostamab) or even CAR-T cells. Indeed, new treatment modalities and data from early phase studies including patients relapsing after CAR-T cell therapy will provide the answer to this challenging problem: "Relapse following BCMA CAR-T cell therapy: hope for further life."

Key Points

- BCMA-directed CAR-T cell therapy shows very encouraging results in triple-class refractory multiple myeloma populations, but there is not yet a survival plateau.
- In the CRB-401 study, an important gap between PFS (median PFS of 8.8 months) and OS (median OS of 34.2 months) was observed, suggesting that patients failing BCMA-directed CAR-T cell therapy may subsequently respond to salvage treatments.
- Data are not yet available to elucidate what optimal rescue therapies should be proposed after CAR-T cell progression.
- Salvage treatments after CAR-T cell treatment should include drugs with new mechanisms of action (i.e., Melflufen, Selinexor, CelMods) or targeting different antigens on the surface of plasma cells (i.e., GPRC5dD (talquetamab) or FcRH5 (cevostamab).

References

Alsina M, Shah N, Raje NS, et al. Updated results from the phase I CRB-402 study of anti-BCMA CAR-T cell therapy bb21217 in patients with relapsed and refractory multiple myeloma: correlation of expansion and duration of response with T cell phenotypes. Blood. 2020;136(Suppl 1):25–6. https://doi.org/10.1182/blood-2020-140410.

Chen L, Xu J, Fu W Sr, et al. Updated phase 1 results of a first-in-human open-label study of Lcar-B38M, a structurally differentiated chimeric antigen receptor T (CAR-T) cell therapy targeting B-cell maturation antigen (BCMA). Blood. 2019;134(Suppl_1):1858. https://doi.org/10.1182/blood-2019-130008.

Cohen AD, Garfall AL, Dogan A, et al. Serial treatment of relapsed/refractory multiple myeloma with different BCMA-targeting therapies. Blood Adv. 2019;3(16):2487–90. https://doi.org/10.1182/bloodadvances.2019000466.

Cohen AD, Hari P, Htut M, et al. Patient expectations and perceptions of treatment in CARTITUDE-1: phase 1b/2 study of ciltacabtagene autoleucel in relapsed/refractory multiple myeloma. Blood. 2020;136(Suppl 1):13–5. https://doi.org/10.1182/blood-2020-136383.

Costello CL, Gregory TK, Ali SA, et al. Phase 2 study of the response and safety of P-BCMA-101 CAR-T cells in patients with relapsed/refractory (r/r) multiple myeloma (MM) (PRIME). Blood. 2019;134(Suppl_1):3184. https://doi.org/10.1182/blood-2019-129562.

D'Agostino M, Raje N. Anti-BCMA CAR-T cell therapy in multiple myeloma: can we do better? Leukemia. 2020;34(1):21–34. https://doi.org/10.1038/s41375-019-0669-4.

Fraietta JA, Lacey SF, Orlando EJ, et al. Determinants of response and resistance to CD19 chimeric antigen receptor (CAR) T cell therapy of chronic lymphocytic leukemia. Nat Med. 2018;24(5):563–71. https://doi.org/10.1038/s41591-018-0010-1.

Gandhi UH, Cornell RF, Lakshman A, et al. Outcomes of patients with multiple myeloma refractory to CD38-targeted monoclonal antibody therapy. Leukemia. 2019;33(9):2266–75. https://doi.org/10.1038/s41375-019-0435-7.

Jiang H, Dong B, Gao L, et al. Clinical results of a multicenter study of the first-in-human dual BCMA and cd19 targeted novel platform fast CAR-T cell therapy for patients with relapsed/refractory multiple myeloma. Blood. 2020;136(Suppl 1):25–6. https://doi.org/10.1182/blood-2020-138614.

Lin Y, Raje NS, Berdeja JG, et al. Idecabtagene vicleucel (ide-cel, bb2121), a BCMA-directed CAR-T cell therapy, in patients with relapsed and refractory multiple myeloma: updated results from Phase 1 CRB-401 study. Blood. 2020;136(Suppl 1):26–7. https://doi.org/10.1182/blood-2020-134324.

Madduri D, Berdeja JG, Usmani SZ, et al. CARTITUDE-1: phase 1b/2 study of ciltacabtagene autoleucel, a B-cell maturation antigen-directed chimeric antigen receptor T cell therapy, in relapsed/refractory multiple myeloma. Blood. 2020;136(Suppl 1):22–5. https://doi.org/10.1182/blood-2020-136307.

Martin T III, Lin Y, Agha M, et al. Health-related quality of life in the cartitude-1 study of ciltacabtagene autoleucel for relapsed/refractory multiple myeloma. Blood. 2020;136(Suppl 1):41–2. https://doi.org/10.1182/blood-2020-136368.

Munshi NC, Anderson LDJ, Shah N, et al. Idecabtagene vicleucel in relapsed and refractory multiple myeloma. N Engl J Med. 2021;384(8):705–16. https://doi.org/10.1056/NEJMoa2024850.

Rodríguez-Otero P, Prósper F, Alfonso A, et al. CAR-T cells in multiple myeloma are ready for prime time. J Clin Med. 2020;9(11) https://doi.org/10.3390/jcm9113577.

Shah N, Delforge M, San-Miguel JF, et al. Secondary quality-of-life domains in patients with relapsed and refractory multiple myeloma treated with the BCMA-directed CAR-T cell therapy idecabtagene vicleucel (ide-cel; bb2121): results from the Karmma clinical trial. Blood. 2020;136(Suppl 1):28–9. https://doi.org/10.1182/blood-2020-136665.

Immune Monitoring

Susanna Carolina Berger, Boris Fehse,
and Marie-Thérèse Rubio

CAR-T cell expansion and persistence are critical parameters for therapeutic efficacy and toxicity (Locke et al. 2020). However, CAR-T cells are patient-specific 'living drugs' with an unpredictable ability to expand in vivo. Thus, close postinfusion monitoring should be a major prerequisite to better manage this therapy. Critical parameters include CAR-T cell expansion kinetics and phenotype immune reconstitution and serum biomarkers (Fig. 35.1; Kalos et al. 2011; Hu and Huang 2020). Additionally, prospective collection and storage of patient specimens should be planned for future hypothesis-driven studies at specialized research centres. To date, despite the rapid expansion of CAR-T cell therapy, no standard recommendations exist for CAR monitoring, and harmonization of efforts across multiple centres is urgently needed.

Molecular Monitoring of CAR-T Cells via Digital PCR (dPCR)

Most clinically used CAR-T cell products consist of autologous lymphocytes stably transduced with retro- or lentiviral vectors encoding the respective CAR construct. Integrated CAR vectors are commonly detected at the genomic level using real-time quantitative PCR (qPCR) or dPCR. Surprisingly, outside of clinical trials, CAR-specific diagnostic tools were initially missing, requiring the de novo design of lab-made specific assays to enumerate CAR-T cells in vivo (Badbaran et al. 2020; Fehse

S. C. Berger (✉) · B. Fehse
Department of Stem Cell Transplantation (SCT) and Research Department Cell and Gene
Therapy, University Medical Center Hamburg-Eppendorf (UKE), Hamburg, Germany
e-mail: su.berger@uke.de; fehse@uke.de

M.-T. Rubio
Service d'Hematolgie, Hôpital Brabois, CHRU Nancy and Biopole de l'Université de
Lorraine, Vandoeuvre les Nancy, France
e-mail: m.rubio@chru-nancy.fr

© The Author(s) 2022
N. Kröger et al. (eds.), *The EBMT/EHA CAR-T Cell Handbook*,
https://doi.org/10.1007/978-3-030-94353-0_35

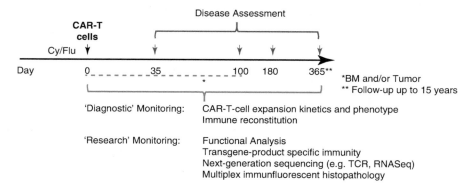

Fig. 35.1 Schematic overview of monitoring after CAR-T cell therapy

et al. 2020; Kunz et al. 2020). Despite technological differences, both qPCR and dPCR assays yield robust and accurate results, with limited requirements regarding sample quality (Table 35.1).

dPCR is extremely sensitive and does not rely on standard curves or multiple repetitions. As a limitation, DNA-directed PCR monitoring provides no information on the expression of the CAR construct. However, the expansion of CAR-T cells strongly depends on the interaction of the CAR with its cognate antigen. In accordance, our data have shown excellent correlation of dPCR with flow cytometry (Badbaran et al. 2020) as well as clinical (Ayuk et al. 2021) results. Because flow cytometry-based assays facilitate phenotypic characterization of CAR-T cells, the two methods complement each other well.

Flow Cytometry Monitoring of CAR-T Cells

Identification of CAR-T cells by flow cytometry (CMF) can be performed by using monoclonal antibodies (mAbs) directly recognizing the CAR (idiotype, linker region) or a specific tag included in the CAR construct. Alternatively, indirect detection can be achieved using antigen-Fc chimeric proteins containing the CAR target antigen fused to a human IgG Fc fragment. A secondary staining step is required for the detection of CAR-expressing cells with an anti-Fc or anti-biotin (if the antigen-Fc is biotinylated) mAb labelled with a fluorochrome (Hu and Huang 2020). In practice, outside of clinical trials, patients receiving commercial CD19 CAR-T cells are monitored with biotinylated CD19-Fc proteins in a two-step staining protocol. The advantage of CMF is the possibility of combining CAR staining with other cell surface markers to characterize CAR-T cells in terms of T cell subtype (CD4 and CD8 expression), differentiation (naïve versus memory), and exhaustion (PD1, TIM3, Lag3). In addition, the results can be provided in real time to physicians. The limitation of the technique is the relatively low sensitivity. Below 0.5% of T cells, the reliability of CMF is weak and justifies pursuing monitoring via PCR. Two important pieces of information can be obtained with sequential CMF analysis of

Table 35.1 Comparison of molecular monitoring tools

	qPCR	dPCR
Principle of analysis		
Target-specific primer and fluorescent probes	Yes	Yes
Analysis of the gene of interest within the sample	At the population level	After partitioning into tiny droplets
Amplification	Amplifies and quantifies amplicon over PCR cycles	Amplifies and quantifies amplicon separately within a droplet
Quantification	Continuous intermediate fluorescence measurements	Relies on end-point fluorescence
Data robustness and reliability	High	Very High[a]
Requirement of a reference sample/standard curve	Yes	No
Single cell tools	No	Yes
Overall properties		
Distribution of the instruments	Commonly available	Still less frequently available
Handling	Easy to implement	Requires more training & technical skills
Cost (Campomenosi et al. 2016)[b]	3.33 € per sample	3.66 € per sample
Multiplexing[c]	Yes	Yes
Certified instruments commercially available?	Yes	Yes (limited)

[a]Compared to qPCR, very robust amplification kinetics and suppresses amplification noise
[b]In the cited study, costs per sample were based on single measurements for dPCR vs. triplicate analyses for qPCR. They did not include instrument amortization
[c]Decreases sample/reagent use and pipetting noise, increases throughput

CAR-T cells in the peripheral blood after cell infusion: the expansion peak (Cmax, maximum CAR-T cell rate in percentage or absolute value) and the area under the curve of circulating CAR-T cells between D0 and D28 (AUC0-28). These two parameters have been associated with the response and the risk of complications after treatment in B-lymphoid malignancies (Park et al. 2018; Fraietta et al. 2018; Locke et al. 2020; Ayuk et al. 2021). To determine these parameters, the recommended frequency of CAR-T cell monitoring is two or three times a week for the first 2 weeks after CAR-T cell administration, on days 21 and 28, once a month until 3 months and then every 3 months until 1 year (Rubio et al. 2021).

Monitoring of Additional Immune Parameters (Non-CAR-T, B, and NK Cells and Cytokines)

Patients receiving anti-CD19 CAR-T cells might develop prolonged T CD4 lymphopenia as well as B-cell aplasia with severe hypogammaglobulinaemia, making them particularly susceptible to bacterial and viral infections even after haematopoietic recovery (Logue et al. 2021). Therefore, routine immune surveillance of non-CAR-T CD4 and CD8 T cells, B cells, and NK cells and the levels of serum immunoglobulins is recommended during the first year of follow-up.

Many cytokines are produced in large quantities after CAR-T cell administration as a result of activation of T lymphocytes (IL-6, IFN-γ, sIL2-Rα, sIL-6R, GM-CSF, IL-2, and TNF-α), activation and attraction of mono-macrophages (IFNα, IL-1β, IL-6, IL1Rα, IL10, IL-12, IL-13, IL-15, sIL6-R, TNF-α, CXCL10, CCL2, and IL-8) and in response to tissue damage (IL-6, IL-8, G-CSF, and GM-CSF) (Brudno and Kochenderfer 2019). Confounding factors, such as sepsis, degree of CAR-T cell expansion and tumour burden, also impact cytokine levels. Some cytokine signatures have been described to predict the occurrence of cytokine release syndrome (CRS) (Teachey et al. 2016), immune effector cell-associated neurotoxicity syndrome (ICANS) (Santomasso et al. 2018) or the expansion capacity of CAR-T cells in vivo (Kochenderfer et al. 2017). One major limitation in clinical practice is the absence of a validated fast cytokine quantification test predicting severe complications. Therefore, further studies are required in homogeneous groups of patients to determine whether cytokines can predict the occurrence of complications or treatment efficacy. Participation in prospective studies or collection of serum at each time point of CAR-T cell analysis is recommended.

Key Points

Immune monitoring after CAR-T cell therapy should be carefully performed:

- Medical CAR-T cell products are complex 'living drugs' with unpredictable in vivo performance. Thus, the establishment of accompanying diagnostic and research monitoring programmes is a priority for rational development of this approach.
- Molecular monitoring, especially dPCR, is an excellent, robust, and sensitive tool for real-time/on-site persistence tracking.
- Flow cytometry is an easy and rapid tool to monitor early CAR-T cell expansion and characterize CAR-T cell phenotype, both of which have been correlated with the response.
- Routine monitoring of T, B, and NK cell populations and immunoglobulin levels is recommended to evaluate infection risk.
- Serum collection is recommended to further explore and identify cytokine signatures that enable prediction of complications or response.
- Efforts to harmonize patient monitoring across multiple centres following CAR-T cell infusion would be desirable (i.e., reference labs, shared databases, and collaborations with dedicated centres for 'next generation' research). Successful implementation of these joint efforts will greatly advance our understanding of the biology involved in transferring CAR-T cells and, most importantly, serve our patients.

References

Ayuk FA, Berger SC, Badbaran A, et al. Axicabtagene ciloleucel in vivo expansion and treatment outcome in aggressive B-cell lymphoma in a real-world setting. Blood Adv. 2021;5(11):2523–7.

Badbaran A, Berger C, Riecken K, et al. Accurate in-vivo quantification of CD19 CAR-T cells after treatment with axicabtagene ciloleucel (Axi-cel) and tisagenlecleucel (Tisa-cel) using digital PCR. Cancers (Basel). 2020;12:1970.

Brudno JN, Kochenderfer JN. Recent advances in CAR-T cell toxicity: mechanisms, manifestations and management. Blood Rev. 2019;34:45–55.

Campomenosi P, Gini E, Noonan DM, et al. A comparison between quantitative PCR and droplet digital PCR technologies for circulating microRNA quantification in human lung cancer. BMC Biotechnol. 2016;16:60.

Fehse B, Badbaran A, Berger C, et al. Digital PCR assays for precise quantification of CD19-CAR-T cells after treatment with axicabtagene ciloleucel. Mol Ther Methods Clin Dev. 2020;16:172–8.

Fraietta JA, Lacey SF, Orlando EJ, et al. Determinants of response and resistance to CD19 chimeric antigen receptor (CAR) T cell therapy of chronic lymphocytic leukemia. Nat Med. 2018;24:563–71.

Hu Y, Huang J. The chimeric antigen receptor detection toolkit. Front Immunol. 2020;11:1770.

Kalos M, Levine BL, Porter DL, et al. T cells with chimeric antigen receptors have potent antitumor effects and can establish memory in patients with advanced leukemia. Sci Transl Med. 2011;3:95ra73.

Kochenderfer JN, Somerville RPT, Lu T, et al. Lymphoma remissions caused by anti-CD19 chimeric antigen receptor T cells are associated with high serum interleukin-15 levels. J Clin Oncol. 2017;35:1803–13.

Kunz A, Gern U, Schmitt A, et al. Optimized assessment of qPCR-based vector copy numbers as a safety parameter for GMP-grade CAR-T cells and monitoring of frequency in patients. Mol Ther Methods Clin Dev. 2020;17:448–54.

Locke FL, Rossi JM, Neelapu SS, et al. Tumor burden, inflammation, and product attributes determine outcomes of axicabtagene ciloleucel in large B-cell lymphoma. Blood Adv. 2020;4:4898–911.

Logue JM, Zucchetti E, Bachmeier CA, et al. Immune reconstitution and associated infections following axicabtagene ciloleucel in relapsed or refractory large B-cell lymphoma. Haematologica. 2021;106(4):978–86.

Park JH, Riviere I, Gonen M, et al. Long-term follow-up of CD19 CAR therapy in acute lymphoblastic leukemia. N Engl J Med. 2018;378:449–59.

Rubio MT, Varlet P, Allain V, et al. Immunomonitoring of patients treated with CAR-T cells for hematological malignancy: guidelines from the CARTi group and the francophone Society of Bone Marrow Transplantation and Cellular Therapy (SFGM-TC). Bull Cancer. 2021;108(12S):S53–64.

Santomasso BD, Park JH, Salloum D, et al. Clinical and biological correlates of neurotoxicity associated with CAR-T cell therapy in patients with B-cell acute lymphoblastic leukemia. Cancer Discov. 2018;8:958–71.

Teachey DT, Lacey SF, Shaw PA, et al. Identification of predictive biomarkers for cytokine release syndrome after chimeric antigen receptor T-cell therapy for acute lymphoblastic leukemia. Cancer Discov. 2016;6:664–79.

Long-Term Follow-Up and Late Effects

36

Patrick Hayden, Nico Gagelmann, and John Snowden

Little is known about the long-term effects of CAR-T cell therapy. Although medium-term complications, such as cytopenia and hypogammaglobulinaemia, may persist and require ongoing treatment, there do not appear to be other durable toxicities specific to this new immunotherapeutic class (Fried et al. 2019; Cordeiro et al. 2020; Cappell et al. 2020). However, to date, CAR-T therapy has been evaluated in patients with multiple relapsed diseases following several lines of treatment, including allogeneic stem cell transplantation, making it difficult to identify which effects may be directly attributable to this novel treatment. Nonetheless, as the use of CAR-T cell therapy increases, structured models for survivorship care will need to be established. The factors that will affect care requirements include the primary malignancy, prior treatment, the specific CAR-T therapy and patient age and frailty.

The main late effects identified to date are shown in Table 36.1. Hypogammaglobulinaemia and prolonged cytopenias appear to be more common in patients with ALL than in patients with B-NHL. In the ELIANA trial, which tested tisagenlecleucel (Kymriah™) in ALL, the median time to B-cell recovery was not reached at a median follow-up time of 13 months (Maude et al. 2018). Prolonged cytopenias in all three cell lines have also been commonly reported. In an Israeli

P. Hayden (✉)
Department of Haematology, Trinity College Dublin, St. James's Hospital, Dublin, Ireland
e-mail: phayden@stjames.ie

N. Gagelmann
Department of Stem Cell Transplantation, University Medical Center Hamburg, Hamburg, Germany
e-mail: n.gagelmann@uke.de

J. Snowden
Department of Haematology, Sheffield Teaching Hospitals NHS Foundation Trust, Sheffield, UK

Department of Oncology and Metabolism, The University of Sheffield, Sheffield, UK
e-mail: john.snowden1@nhs.net

© The Author(s) 2022
N. Kröger et al. (eds.), *The EBMT/EHA CAR-T Cell Handbook*,
https://doi.org/10.1007/978-3-030-94353-0_36

Table 36.1 Main late effects after CAR-T cell therapy

Effect	Occurrence	Management
Cytopenia (esp. neutropenia) All grades >2	Two months after infusion: ~50% ~20%	Transfusion, growth factors, infection prophylaxis
Hypogammaglobulinaemia	~50%, prolonged years after infusion	Intravenous immunoglobulins (IVIGs)
Infections	Predominantly upper respiratory tract, >50% bacterial	IVIGs, antibiotics, viral screening, vaccination
Secondary malignancies	Solid tumour > haematological	Surveillance, awareness
Neurological effects	~10%, neuropathy and cerebrovascular events	Supportive care, interdisciplinary approach to diagnosis and therapy
Psychiatric issues	~10%, depression and anxiety	
Immune-related issues	<10%, alveolitis, pneumonitis, dermatitis, arthralgia, and myositis, etc.	Corticosteroids, immunosuppression, interdisciplinary approach to diagnosis and therapy

study of 29 patients with either ALL or B-NHL responding after treatment with CTL109 with a CD28 costimulatory domain, factors associated with late cytopenias were prior allo-HCT and higher-grade CRS (Fried et al. 2019).

Apart from one patient in the ZUMA-1 trial who developed MDS at 19 months, there were no secondary malignancies reported in the three clinical trials that led to licensing of CD-19-directed therapy in B-ALL and B-NHL. In addition, some late cancers are to be expected in such heavily pretreated patients. Although there is one report of unintended insertion of the CAR gene into leukaemic B cells, thus far, there have been no reports of insertional oncogenesis during CAR-T cell production.

The role of vaccinations following CAR-T cell therapy remains unclear. Until evidence-based specific CAR-T vaccination programmes are produced, protocols similar to HSCT should be considered (Majhail et al. 2012).

Follow-Up and Programmes

As a specialized service, CAR-T therapy in Europe is generally provided based on a hub-and-spoke model: patients are referred from local hospitals to regional cellular therapy centres. One option is to provide follow-up in JACIE-accredited allo-HCT late effects clinics alongside transplant recipients. They operate on a checklist model to ensure that survivors are systematically and longitudinally assessed for late toxicities. Over time, dedicated CAR-T late effects clinics can be developed if the growing pool of survivors reaches a critical mass. Service-level agreements (SLAs) between CAR-T centres and referral centres should cover shared care and outreach arrangements.

Such clinics require multidisciplinary team (MDT) input, including physicians involved in CAR-T administration, clinical nurse specialists, clinical psychologists, data managers, and clinical trial staff. All CAR-T recipients will have been heavily pretreated. Therefore, a cumulative burden of broader physical and psychological late effects will need to be considered. Areas to cover in the clinic include CAR-T persistence; secondary malignancies; autoimmune disease; endocrine, reproductive and bone health; psychological health; and patient-reported outcomes, including quality of life (Buitrago et al. 2019; Ruark et al. 2020). Importantly, the patient-reported quality-of-life studies performed thus far indicate levels of physical and mental health comparable to that in the normal population.

Initial follow-up will be determined by the status of the underlying disease. Patients should be seen monthly for the first year, when the focus will be on remission status alongside any short-term complications. Subsequent follow-up can focus on longer-term effects, 6 months for the following 2 years, annually until the 15 year, and potentially indefinitely. Patients who proceed to subsequent HSCT, cytotoxic therapy and/or immune effector cell therapy should be followed as recommended by Majhail et al. (2012).

Post-authorisation Safety Surveillance (PASS)

As both tisagenlecleucel (Kymriah™) and axicabtagene ciloleucel (Yescarta™) are based on genetic modification of autologous T-cells using viral vectors, the EMA and FDA made marketing approval conditional on a 15-year PASS. In 2019, the cellular therapy module of the EBMT registry was found by the EMA to be fit-for-purpose for regulatory oversight of such pharmacoepidemiological studies. The MED-A cell therapy form has been modified for use with CAR-T cells and other academic- or industry-manufactured cell therapies. In November 2020, the German health insurance regulator directed centres to report commercial CAR-T cell treatments to the EBMT Registry and confirmed that reporting such data will be a condition for reimbursement of the costs of CAR-T cell therapy.

JACIE

FACT-JACIE standards were initially developed for the accreditation of HCT programmes (Snowden et al. 2017; Saccardi et al. 2019). The current seventh edition of the standards also covers immune effector cells (IECs) to accommodate cellular therapy, including CAR-T cells. In addition to clauses addressing the need for policies on the management of acute toxicities, standard B.7.12 specifies the need for "policies and Standard Operating Procedures for monitoring by appropriate specialists of recipients for post-cellular therapy late effects". Inspection of IEC standards is incorporated within standard JACIE site visits.

For centres that undertake CAR-T cell therapy outside of an accredited allo-HCT programme, there are a number of options. Given that most CAR-T cell therapies are currently used to treat lymphoma, compliance with the IEC standards can be achieved as part of the accreditation covering autologous HCT (auto-HCT). The same considerations could apply to myeloma specialists working outside of allo-HCT programmes. In the event of CAR-T cells or related therapies becoming applicable more broadly to nonhaematological cancers, an alternative strategy already adopted by FACT is to undertake independent IEC accreditation specifically for CAR-T cells and other IECs. JACIE also provides a robust method to ensure that programmes meet the requirements for mandatory long-term data submission to the EBMT Registry, as well as potential benchmarking of survival outcomes.

The eighth edition of the FACT-JACIE standards will be published in 2021 with more detail on immune effector cells to help provide a framework for centres to establish and assure the quality and safe practice of treatment administration and short- and long-term follow-up of CAR-T therapy.

Key Points
- To date, few durable toxicities have been directly attributable to CAR-T cell therapy.
- The principal late effects identified to date include hypogammaglobulinaemia, cytopenias, and infections.
- Structured models for survivorship care include JACIE-accredited allo-HCT late effects clinics.
- Areas to monitor in the clinic include CAR-T persistence; secondary malignancies; autoimmune disease; endocrine, reproductive and bone health; psychological health; and patient-reported outcomes, including quality of life.
- EMA has mandated 15-year postauthorization safety surveillance (PASS) of all CAR-T cell therapies, and the cellular therapy module of the EBMT registry has been approved for this purpose.
- The current seventh edition of the FACT-JACIE transplant standards also covers immune effector cells (IECs) to accommodate cellular therapy, including CAR-T cells.

References

Buitrago J, Adkins S, Hawkins M, Iyamu K, Oort T. Adult survivorship: considerations following CAR-T cell therapy. Clin J Oncol Nurs. 2019;23(2):42–8.

Cappell KM, Sherry RM, Yang JC, Goff SL, Vanasse DA, McIntyre L, et al. Long-term follow-up of anti-cd19 chimeric antigen receptor T-cell therapy. J Clin Oncol. 2020;38(32):3805–15.

Cordeiro A, Bezerra ED, Hirayama AV, Hill JA, Wu QV, Voutsinas J, et al. Late events after treatment with CD19-targeted chimeric antigen receptor modified T cells. Biol Blood Marrow Transplant. 2020;26(1):26–33.

Fried S, Avigdor A, Bielorai B, Meir A, Besser MJ, Schachter J, et al. Early and late hematologic toxicity following CD19 CAR-T cells. Bone Marrow Transplant. 2019;54(10):1643–50.

Majhail NS, Rizzo JD, Lee SJ, Aljurf M, Atsuta Y, Bonfim C, et al. Recommended screening and preventive practices for long-term survivors after hematopoietic cell transplantation. Bone Marrow Transplant. 2012;47(3):337–41.

Maude SL, Laetsch TW, Buechner J, Rives S, Boyer M, Bittencourt H, et al. Tisagenlecleucel in children and young adults with B-cell lymphoblastic leukemia. N Engl J Med. 2018;378(5):439–48.

Ruark J, Mullane E, Cleary N, Cordeiro A, Bezerra ED, Wu V, et al. Patient-reported neuropsychiatric outcomes of long-term survivors after chimeric antigen receptor T cell therapy. Biol Blood Marrow Transplant. 2020;26(1):34–43.

Saccardi R, McGrath E, Snowden AJ. JACIE accreditation of HSCT programs. In: The EBMT handbook; 2019. p. 35–40.

Snowden JA, McGrath E, Duarte RF, Saccardi R, Orchard K, Worel N, et al. JACIE accreditation for blood and marrow transplantation: past, present and future directions of an international model for healthcare quality improvement. Bone Marrow Transplant. 2017;52(10):1367–71.

Part V
Access to CAR-T Cells

The Regulatory Framework for CAR-T Cells in Europe: Current Status and Foreseeable Changes AND Centre Qualification by Competent Authorities and Manufacturers

Eoin McGrath and Petr Machalik

Current Framework

Under current European Union regulations, CAR-T cell therapies fall under the advanced therapy medicinal products (ATMPs) framework. ATMPs represent a category of medicinal products defined in EU Regulation 1394/2007 and subdivided into four categories, of which autologous or allogeneic CAR-T cells, among other therapies, are considered gene therapy medicinal products (GTMPs). ATMPs are subject to a centralized evaluation framework whereby one authorization is valid for all countries in the EU led by the European Medicines Agency's Committee for Advanced Therapies (CAT). The framework includes different regulatory pathways for bringing ATMPs from clinical trials to market authorization, and the regulatory pathway taken will depend on a product's characteristics and the target patient population. In 2018, two chimeric antigen receptor (CAR) T cell therapies, Yescarta and Kymriah, completed their authorization process via the priority medicines PRIME scheme to Marketing Authorization (Detela and Lodge 2019).

The production, distribution, and administration of ATMPs require a completely different organization plan than that used for HSCT, with manufacturing typically at a central facility in compliance with good manufacturing practices (GMPs), a version of which was released in 2017 by the European Commission to specifically

E. McGrath
EBMT, Barcelona, Spain
e-mail: eoin.mcgrath@ebmt.org

P. Machalik (✉)
Be The Match BioTherapies, Minneapolis, MN, USA
e-mail: pmachali@nmdp.org

deal with the manufacturing of ATMPs.[1] Since a majority of the ATMPs that progress to authorization or at least to clinical trials are manufactured from autologous mononuclear cells, starting material is usually procured by hospital- or blood bank-operated apheresis facilities, creating a peculiar situation in which a product starts under one regulation—EU Tissues and Cells Directives[2]—before passing to another—ATMP Regulation- and in which a hospital acts as a service provider to industry, an interaction that requires further definition of the respective responsibilities and liabilities (McGrath and Chabannon 2018). The Tissues and Cells Directives, which cover all steps in the transplant process from donation, procurement, testing, processing, preservation, storage, and distribution, are undergoing a review that is expected to lead to a legislative proposal by the European Commission in late 2021, and it is anticipated that the new framework will further consider how products cross the interface between the two frameworks.

Given the high toxicity profile of CAR-T cell therapies, marketing authorization may be subject to conditions that lead to a risk management plan (RMP). The RMP for the currently authorized CAR-T therapies includes the need for manufacturers to qualify the sites that will treat patients. Site qualification is addressed below.

Hospital Exemption

In recognizing that many potential ATMPs are used for limited numbers of patients and with little commercial interest, Regulation 1394/2007 created the so-called hospital exemption (HE) under Article 28, exempting from authorization requirements those ATMPs manufactured in hospitals or universities where the medicine is prescribed for individual patients under the care of a medical practitioner. This manufacturing should occur on a nonroutine basis according to specific quality standards (GMPs) and only within the same member state.

In February 2021, the Spanish pharmaceutical regulator AEMPS authorized the first CAR-T cell therapy approved by a European national authority under the hospital exemption clause for the ARI-0001 CAR-T developed by the Hospital Clinic in Barcelona.[3]

National authorities oversee the approval of HE products, which has resulted in significant variations between member states in how approval is applied, in turn leading to criticism from both industry and academia that the approval process is unclear and inconsistent.

---

[1] Guidelines of 22.11.2017 Good Manufacturing Practice for Advanced Therapy Medicinal Products. EudraLex The Rules Governing Medicinal Products in the European Union Volume 4 Good Manufacturing Practice.

[2] Directive 2004/23 of the European Parliament and of the Council of 31 March 2004 on setting standards of quality and safety for the donation, procurement, testing, processing, preservation, storage, and distribution of human tissues and cells.

[3] https://www.aemps.gob.es/informa/notasinformativas/medicamentosusohumano-3/2021-medicamentosusohumano-3/la-aemps-autoriza-el-car-t-ari-0001-del-hospital-clinic-para-pacientes-con-leucemia-linfoblastica-aguda/?lang=en. Accessed 13/03/2021.

Role of Academia

Academia remains very active in the early phases of clinical trials designed to evaluate innovative GTMPs as potential complements, substitutes, or bridges to historical forms of haematopoietic cell transplants. One recent study calculated that even now, when industry interest in these therapies has increased significantly in the last 5–6 years, over 50% of CAR-T cell trials in the USA are still sponsored by academia (Kassir et al. 2020). Many public institutions have invested significant resources to upgrade their processing facilities to GMP-compliant levels, thus allowing for small-scale manufacturing of experimental medicinal products to support phase I and possibly phase II studies. Furthermore, academia must become a proactive stakeholder in the regulatory area by engaging with the authorities, sharing their know-how and voicing their opinion. Through continental registries, such as EBMT, academic institutions will continue to play a key role due to their data and procedural knowledge, which will be very useful not only for researchers but also for industry, health care regulators and payers (Hildebrandt 2020).

Health Technology Assessment

For a marketing authorization holder, approval by EMA is just one step. To gain market access in the EU, the manufacturer must now approach national health care reimbursement authorities, collectively known as health technology assessment (HTA) bodies, who will assess the cost of the added value of novel therapies compared to the current standard of care. Unlike the centralized authorization process, HTA assessments are performed at the national level and are subject to great variability between member states. Over the past decade, the EU has pursued a more harmonized HTA process across Europe, although there remains significant resistance among member states, and a legislative proposal adopted by the Commission in early 2018 is only very slowly progressing through the parliamentary process.

Future Focus

Access to ATMPs, including cellular therapies, is likely to be a particular challenge for patients, health care professionals, and national health systems due to their expected high costs and complexity. Foreseeable changes to the regulatory framework could see closer alignment with MA and HTA to make them more concurrent and less sequential processes. The EMA's strategy for big data places an emphasis on using real-world data (RWD) to support regulatory decisions, and significant efforts are being made to prepare the structures to support this move. Accelerated processes, such as PRIME, will continue to evolve as regulators gain more knowledge and the science and medicine develop. The interplay between European medicinal product regulations and genetically modified organism (GMO) frameworks will likely continue to be the focus of efforts to harmonize interpretations across the EU. Regulators will see more automation of manufacturing processes, which should help reduce risk and variability, while decentralized or 'bedside' manufacturing could become more common but still need regulatory approval and oversight. Allogeneic CAR-T products will also require substantial evidence to reassure regulators regarding safety concerns about graft versus host disease, cell rejection, and the risks associated with gene editing. Data protection measures under the General Data Protection Regulation (GDPR) for health-related personal data could see adaptations to better facilitate secondary use of data collected to support investigational and regulatory needs.

Centre Qualification by Competent Authorities and Manufacturers

Shared Goals

A high degree of competencies is required from centres involved in CAR-T cell therapies by both the competent authorities and the manufacturers. With regard to centre qualification, authorities and manufacturers share at least some own goals, which is minimizing CAR-T cell therapy-associated risks for patients to deliver safe and efficient therapy. Authorities at the international, national, or regional levels assess the quality of care, level of practice and health outcomes, and qualify centres that successfully demonstrate high standards of health care and patient safety. For a manufacturer, accreditation by the competent authority verifies that the required standards are followed and the necessary qualifications, processes and resources are present. From the centre's perspective, receiving necessary accreditations and approvals from both the competent authority and the respective manufacturer is a prerequisite to support concrete CAR-T cell therapy.

Centre Assessment

The presence of accreditation by a competent authority is among the first items checked by a manufacturer during the so-called feasibility assessment. The other reviewed items include the scope of authorized activities; the centre's ability to perform particular procedures and tests, incorporate the manufacturer's requirements, and guarantee specific environmental conditions; and the presence of requested equipment and qualified personnel. For a manufacturer, the assessment is a great chance to obtain a better understanding of a centre's setup and daily routine and its procedural and capacity constraints. The assessment might also reveal gaps, such as the inadequateness or complete absence of required processes. Generally, the feasibility assessment is a unique opportunity to evaluate prospective candidates for collaboration, and it precedes all other steps in a centre's qualification by a manufacturer, which may vary in scope and detail depending on the particular therapy.

Centre Auditing

The centre qualification audit is usually performed by a manufacturer prior to commencement of any collaboration. The aim is to evaluate compliance with applicable regulatory requirements and the centre's own procedures or policies. Manufacturers obtain an appropriate understanding of the performed services and the robustness of engaged systems, including quality management, personnel training, and the capacity of available resources. They usually request some of the centre's internal documents and process details to be shared prior to the audit to allow for a thorough review. During the audit, auditors examine more of the centre's documentation, interview personnel, inspect the facility's key locations, and evaluate processes in targeted functional areas.

In the course of an established collaboration, other types of audits can be organized. The so-called surveillance audit is a periodic audit to ensure that a centre is continuing to comply with the required standards. The emphasis is on reviewing significant changes that have occurred in the relevant procedures, facility and its quality system since the qualification audit. A follow-up on any previous audit findings, including the implementation of corrective and preventive actions, is also a common part of surveillance audits, which are usually performed every 2–3 years.

A for-cause audit can be called in response to serious circumstances, including deficiency in meeting regulatory requirements, occurrence of a major deviation, repeated deviations, or the risk or occurrence of patient safety issues. This audit generally focuses on identified nonconformities and areas of manufacturer concern.

Any type of audit will result in an audit report, which lists audit observations or findings that might be evaluated for significance as minor, major, or critical. In response to a finding, a centre's own internal procedure usually mandates insurance of a corrective action. This frequently means strengthening the existing processes or creation of brand-new processes. Acceptable responses to audit findings are required to close an audit.

Centre Training

Audited centres are further qualified by the manufacturers for support of concrete CAR-T cell therapy. Manufacturers usually do not aim to boost personnel's general knowledge or the skills and attitudes required for daily routine practice. Their focus is on explaining the specificities of clinical trials or authorized therapies, with few differences between the requirements of the two categories. Generally, the critical parameters of procedures and products are explained, as well as timelines, environmental conditions, types of equipment and material, completion and usage of involved documents, and principles of communication among stakeholders. Due to the complexity of CAR-T cell therapies, centre personnel qualified by manufacturers perform a wide range of functions. Manufacturers usually train those involved in patient or donor care; starting material procurement, processing, intermediate storage, packaging, release, and testing; completion of documents; and ATMP receipt, storage, thawing and administration. In practice, these functions involve physicians, nurses, pharmacists, apheresis and laboratory technicians, and administrative workers.

Required procedure parameters include duration limits, processed volume targets, type of anticoagulant, environmental conditions (such as temperature and humidity), and methods of disconnecting and sealing collection bags. Product parameters that manufacturers like to specify include targets for collected volume, yield and purity and the required number of units and samples. With regard to timelines, the importance of procedure scheduling and harmonization with other procedural steps or treatment sessions is emphasized. Manufacturers are usually very clear about the type of equipment and material required for procurement, intermediate storage, indoor transport, the processing and packaging of starting material or storage, and thawing and administration of ATMPs. The purpose and usage of the involved documents are explained, and instructions for completing, archiving, or sharing with other stakeholders are provided. Colour-coded sample documents, prepopulated forms, and checklists are among the most frequent support materials.

Centre qualification is not bound to its on-site execution. It can also be performed remotely when travel or visitor restrictions or social distancing guidelines make any externally driven on-site activities impossible. Internet-based applications, teleconferencing tools, and purposely developed virtual procedures have recently been successfully used by manufacturers to perform feasibility assessments, audits, and trainings.

Key Points
- CAR-T cell therapy falls under the ATMP framework, presenting challenges to all stakeholders, including health care providers and patients.
- Regulatory issues concern not only marketing authorization but also mechanisms for cost–benefit assessment and, less directly, GMOs and data protection.
- Academia will continue to play a significant role in the development and delivery of these new therapies and should expect to engage with other stakeholders.
- The regulatory framework is not static and evolves with experience and knowledge.
- Competent authorities and manufacturers have a common goal, which is minimizing CAR-T cell therapy-associated risks for patients.
- Accreditation of a centre by a competent authority is understood as verification that the required standards are followed and the necessary qualifications, processes and resources are present.
- Manufacturers qualify centres for support of a concrete CAR-T cell therapy and focus on the specificities of a particular project.
- Centre qualification is not bound to on-site execution and can be performed remotely using internet-based applications, teleconferencing tools, and purposely developed virtual procedures.

Sources of Information

- World Health Organization—Patient Safety [Internet]. 13 September 2019. Available from: https://www.who.int/news-room/fact-sheets/detail/patient-safety (Accessed February 2021)
- Yakoub-Agha I, Chabannon C, Bader P, Basak GW, Bonig H, Ciceri F, Corbacioglu S, Duarte RF, Einsele H, Hudecek M, Kernsten MJ, Köhl U, Kuball J, Mielke S, Mohty M, Murray J, Nagler A, Robinson S, Saccardi R, Sanchez-Guijo F, Snowden JA, Srour M, Styczynski J, Urbano-Ispizua A, Hayden PJ, Kröger N. Management of adults and children undergoing chimeric antigen receptor T-cell therapy: best practice recommendations of the European Society for Blood and Marrow Transplantation (EBMT) and the Joint Accreditation Committee of ISCT and EBMT (JACIE) [Internet]. February 2020. Available from: https://haematologica.org/article/view/9515 (Accessed February 2021)
- Taylor L, Rodriguez ES, Reese A, Anderson K. Building a Program—Implications for infrastructure, nursing education, and training for CAR-T cell therapy. Clin J Oncol Nurs. 2019 Apr 1;23(2):20–26. https://doi.org/10.1188/19.CJON.S1.20-26. [Internet]. Available from: https://pubmed.ncbi.nlm.nih.gov/30880820/ (Accessed February 2021)
- Black A, Gabriel S, Caulfield D. Implementing chimeric antigen receptor T-cell therapy in practice. The Pharmaceutical Journal [Internet]. 22 May 2020. Available from: https://pharmaceutical-journal.com/article/ld/implementing-chimeric-antigen-receptor-t-cell-therapy-in- practice (Accessed February 2021)
- **Quality System Audit Program—Activate apheresis and cell collection sites faster by licensing GTP audit results. Be The Match BioTherapies. [Internet]. Available from: https://bethematchbiotherapies.com/solutions/quality--system-audit-program/ (Accessed February 2021)**
- **Vincinis R. Major vs. Minor Audit Findings. The Auditor. [Internet]. Available from: https://www.theauditoronline.com/major-vs-minor-audit-findings/ (Accessed February 2021)**

References

Detela G, Lodge A. EU regulatory pathways for ATMPs: standard, accelerated and adaptive pathways to marketing authorisation. Mol Therap Method Clin Develop. 2019;13:205–32. https://doi.org/10.1016/j.omtm.2019.01.010.

Hildebrandt M. Horses for courses: an approach to the qualification of clinical trial sites and investigators in ATMPs. Drug Discov Today. 2020;25(2):265–8. https://doi.org/10.1016/j.drudis.2019.10.003.

Kassir Z, et al. Sponsorship and funding for gene therapy trials in the United States. JAMA Am Med Assoc. 2020;323(9):890. https://doi.org/10.1001/jama.2019.22214.

McGrath E, Chabannon C. Regulatory aspects of ATMP versus minimally manipulated immune cells. In: The EBMT handbook: hematopoietic stem cell transplantation and cellular therapies. Springer; 2018. p. 461–4. https://doi.org/10.1007/978-3-030-02278-5_62.

How Can Accreditation Bodies, Such as JACIE or FACT, Support Centres in Getting Qualified?

Riccardo Saccardi and Fermin Sanchez-Guijo

The FACT-JACIE accreditation system is based on a standard-driven process covering all the steps of HSC transplant activity, from donor selection to clinical care. Since the first approval of the First Edition of the Standards in 1998, over 360 HSCT programmes or facilities have been accredited at least once, most of them achieving subsequent re-accreditations (Snowden et al. 2017). The positive impact of the accreditation process in the EBMT Registry has been well established (Gratwohl et al. 2014). Starting with version 6.1, the standards include new items specifically developed for other cellular therapy products, with special reference to immune effector cells (IECs). This reflects the rapid evolution of the field of cellular therapy, primarily (but not exclusively) through the use of genetically modified cells, such as CAR-T cells. FACT-JACIE standards cover a wide range of important aspects that can be of use for centres that aim to be accredited in their countries to provide IEC therapy. Notably, FACT-JACIE accreditation itself is a key (or even a prerequisite) condition in some countries for approval by health authorities to provide commercial CAR-T cell therapy and is also valued by pharmaceutical companies (both those developing clinical trials and those manufacturing commercial products), which also inspect the cell therapy programmes and facilities established at each centre (Hayden et al. 2021). Interest in applying for FACT-JACIE accreditation that includes IEC therapeutic programmes is clearly increasing, from four applications in 2017 to 36 applications approved in 2019. The standards do not cover the manufacturing of such cells but include the chain of responsibilities when the product is

R. Saccardi
Cell Therapy and Transfusion Medicine Unit, Careggi University Hospital, Florence, Italy
e-mail: riccardo.saccardi@aouc.unifi.it

F. Sanchez-Guijo (✉)
Cell Therapy Area and Hematology Department, University Hospital of Salamanca, Salamanca, Spain

Department of Medicine, University of Salamanca, Salamanca, Spain
e-mail: ferminsg@usal.es

provided by a third party (Maus and Nikiforow 2017). In any case, all the steps in the process in which the centre is involved (e.g., patient or donor evaluations, cell collection, cell reception, and storage) are covered by the standards, including the appropriate agreements with the internal partners, including the pharmacy department. In addition, from a clinical perspective, IECs may require special safety monitoring systems due to the high frequency of acute adverse events related to the massive immunological reaction against the tumour. Although examples and explanations are found in the standard manual, here, the special importance of identifying and managing cytokine release syndrome (CRS) should be emphasized, and the standards focus not on specific therapeutic algorithms but on ensuring that medical and nursing teams are sufficiently trained in the early detection of this and other potential complications (e.g., neurological complications). They also pay attention to the full-time availability within the institution and its pharmacy of the necessary medication to address complications and the capacitation and involvement of Intensive Care and Neurology Department professionals to provide urgent care if needed. Forthcoming cellular therapy products, currently under investigation, will show a wider range of risk profiles, therefore requiring product-specific risk assessment and consequent adaptation of the clinical procedures for different classes of products. The FACT-JACIE standards will continue to adapt to these future needs to assist centres in their achievement of optimal clinical outcomes.

Key Points
- FACT-JACIE standards have helped accredited centres improve their HSCT clinical outcomes for more than 20 years.
- Standards have been adapted to cover immune effector cell (IEC) therapy and are a key element in demonstrating optimal quality and performance for seeking accreditation by both National Health Authorities and the pharmaceutical companies involved.
- The IEC product chain of responsibilities, agreements with all involved partners, and full coverage of related adverse events are among the key elements of IEC-related standards.

References

Gratwohl A, Brand R, McGrath E, et al. Use of the quality management system "JACIE" and outcome after hematopoietic stem cell transplantation. Haematologica. 2014;99:908–15.

Hayden PJ, Roddie C, Bader P, Basak GW, Bonig H, Bonini C, et al. Management of adults and children receiving CAR T-cell therapy: 2021 best practice recommendations of the European Society for Blood and Marrow Transplantation (EBMT) and the Joint Accreditation Committee of ISCT and EBMT (JACIE) and the European Haematology Association (EHA). Ann Oncol. 2021;S0923–7534(21):04876–6. https://doi.org/10.1016/j.annonc.2021.12.003. Online ahead of print.

Maus MV, Nikiforow S. The why, what, and how of the new FACT standards for immune effector cells. J Immunother Cancer. 2017;5:36.

Snowden JA, McGrath E, Duarte RF, et al. JACIE accreditation for blood and marrow transplantation: past, present and future directions of an international model for healthcare quality improvement. Bone Marrow Transplant. 2017;52:1367–71.

Educational Needs for Physicians

Nicolaus Kröger ⓘ, John Gribben ⓘ, and Isabel Sánchez-Ortega

CAR-T cells are novel therapies associated with promising and potentially curative outcomes in patients with high-risk relapsed disease. In Europe, there are currently three approved products (tisagenlecleucel, axicabtagene ciloleucel, and brexucabtagene autoleucel) for patients with acute lymphoblastic leukaemia, aggressive B-cell lymphoma, and mantle cell lymphoma, although expanded haematologic and non-haematologic indications are expected soon.

Cellular therapy, including CAR-T cells, is a rapidly evolving field in haematology, and treatment is becoming personalized and specific. To ensure optimal decision-making by physicians, adequate education programmes must be available and must be regularly updated. There is a need to identify knowledge gaps and barriers to address these issues with continuous medical education. Adequate education increases the competence and performance of physicians and improves the quality of decision-making, ultimately resulting in the optimization of patient management. The importance of education is also reflected in the JACIE accreditation scheme, the major objective of which is to promote quality medical and laboratory practice in cellular therapy by offering accreditation based on internationally recognized standards. The relevant standards in this scheme require that clinical, collection, and processing facility staff participate in continuous education activities (JACIE 2021). However, there is also a need to educate the wider community (people who do not

N. Kröger (✉)
Department of Stem Cell Transplantation, University Medical Center Hamburg-Eppendorf, Hamburg, Germany
e-mail: nkroeger@uke.de

J. Gribben
Bart's Cancer Institute, Queen Mary University of London, London, UK
e-mail: j.gribben@qmul.ac.uk

I. Sánchez-Ortega
EBMT, Executive Office, Barcelona, Spain
e-mail: isabel.sanchez-ortega@ebmt.org

© The Author(s) 2022
N. Kröger et al. (eds.), *The EBMT/EHA CAR-T Cell Handbook*,
https://doi.org/10.1007/978-3-030-94353-0_39

work at JACIE accredited sites) to ensure sufficient knowledge to recognize the role of CAR-T therapy, identify suitable patients and understand the process for timely referral to treatment centres. There is an inevitable delay between referral, cell collection, and delivery of the CAR-T products, and physicians must be aware of this process and take steps to manage their patients, who are at high risk of rapid disease progression and may require bridging therapy, ideally in close collaboration with the CAR-T treatment centre. Therefore, referring physicians must be educated to understand the patient selection process, T cell collection process, and the processing and conditioning therapy to fully understand the path that their patients will travel and the time frames involved in delivering these complex treatments.

CAR-T cell therapies are associated with remarkable therapeutic response rates but also with unique and potentially lethal complications that require specific educational updates. Cytokine-release syndrome (CRS) and neurotoxicity are the most frequent complications after CAR-T cell therapies. These complications can occur concomitantly and may have a very rapid onset, with a spectrum of symptoms that range from mild to life threatening. In addition, CRS onset is often indistinguishable from infection, which, in the setting of neutropenia, makes the management of these complex patients even more challenging (Hayden et al. 2021). Haematologic toxicity, most often seen as a complication of lymphodepleting induction therapy, is frequent after CAR-T cell infusion, but the pattern, duration, and outcome are not well described. Learning to monitor and adequately treat persistent cytopenias is necessary for adequate management of these patients. Learning to define the optimal timing for ICU referral is also critical because any delay in ICU admission can compromise patient outcomes. In addition, the unique toxicity profile of CAR-T cell therapies makes incorporation of real-life data, including that from the patients' perspective, essential, and initial data suggest that patient-reported toxicities and mental health concerns are common throughout all stages of survivorship (Barata et al. 2021; Hoogland et al. 2021). From the moment that a patient is identified as a CAR-T candidate, education and supportive care of patients undergoing CAR-T therapy is crucial to improve the knowledge and experience of the patients and their families. To address these issues, a trained multidisciplinary team, including haematologists, oncologists, intensivists, neurologists, pharmacists, psychologists, and nurses, must work together from the time of potential patient identification to the time of treatment and discharge, and their roles are crucial at different stages in the CAR-T cell process.

Large registry studies with high-quality data may provide the basis of knowledge for CAR-T cell therapies and open the door to the necessary specific subpopulation investigations. To ensure continuous evaluation of the efficacy and safety of commercially available CAR-T cells, the EMA endorsed the use of the EBMT registry for collection of 15-year follow-up data of treated patients (EMA 2019). Likewise, follow-up data of patients receiving academic and other pharmaceutical-sponsored CAR-T cell therapies are also expected to be reported to the EBMT registry. Therefore, the real-world data contained in the EBMT registry will likely be a major source of knowledge to improve the use of CAR-T cell therapies and to understand the short-term and long-term patient toxicities and outcomes. This will also allow us to gain insights into potential biomarkers and the patient and disease characteristics that might impact the efficacy of CAR-T-treatment, opening the path to more effective selection and stratification of patients.

Ongoing investigations of CAR-T cell therapies are seeking to elucidate the mechanisms of resistance, immune escape, and relapse so that the current barriers can be overcome and treatment efficacy can be improved. Research is also focused on access to "off-the-shelf" allogeneic CAR-T products, simplifying the manufacturing process and mitigating side effects, among other aims. Thus, the complexity and rapid changes in the field of cellular therapies demands wide collaboration to maintain up-to-date education on the entire pathway from collection to the manufacturer and back to the clinical unit. GoCART, a multistakeholder coalition launched by EBMT and EHA, offers a platform to provide the required diversified and topic-specific education on CAR-T cell therapies. Likewise, the annual EBMT/EHA European CAR-T cell meeting provides specific continuous medical education in this complex field. In addition, educational online updates are provided on the EBMT and EHA e-learning platforms (https://www.ebmt.org/education/e--learning, https://ehacampus.ehaweb.org) with specific webinars and e-learning courses focused not only on CAR-T cells but also on other evolving immunotherapy treatments that may impact the pathway towards CAR-T cell treatment. There is still much to learn, and this rapidly evolving field requires rapid and constant educational updates.

Key Points
- Continuous medical education should fill unavoidable knowledge gaps in a rapidly evolving field.
- Big data registry studies, multistakeholder coalitions, and multidisciplinary educational meetings provide regular updates on the entire CAR-T cell therapy process.
- Updates on specific topics and the latest scientific developments are also required to provide individualized high-quality patient management.
- e-learning platforms and CAR-T cell meetings provide adequate and specific updates in this complex field, but there is also a need to educate the wider medical community, who refer patients to treatment centres.
- Continuous medical education is necessary, especially because this field is rapidly evolving.

References

Barata A, Hoogland A, Hyland K, et al. Patient-reported toxicities in axicabtagene ciloleucel recipients: 1-year follow-up. Transpl Cell Therap. 2021;27(3):S375. https://doi.org/10.1016/S2666-6367(21)00485-1.

EMA qualification opinion on cellular therapy module of the EBMT Registry. 2019. Available at: https://www.ema.europa.eu/en/cellular-therapy-module-european-society-blood-marrow-transplantation-ebmt-registry.

Hayden PJ, Roddie C, Bader P, Basak GW, Bonig H, Bonini C, et al. Management of adults and children receiving CAR T-cell therapy: 2021 best practice recommendations of the European Society for Blood and Marrow Transplantation (EBMT) and the Joint Accreditation Committee of ISCT and EBMT (JACIE) and the European Haematology Association (EHA). Ann Oncol. 2021;S0923–7534(21):04876–6. https://doi.org/10.1016/j.annonc.2021.12.003. Online ahead of print.

Hoogland A, Jayani R, Collier A, et al. Acute patient-reported outcomes in B-cell malignancies treated with axicabtagene ciloleucel. Cancer Med. 2021;10(6):1936–43.

JACIE. 2021. Available at: https://www.ebmt.org/accreditation/jacie-standards.

Education Needs for Nurses in Adult and Paediatric Units

40

Michelle Kenyon, John Murray, Rose Ellard, and Daphna Hutt

Complex nursing care for patients on the CAR-T cell therapy pathway involves many different nursing roles that have important functions at different stages in the pathway. Within the multiprofessional team, nurse education is critical to safe and competent care and to the patient's treatment experience. As we consider the education needs of the nursing workforce throughout the entire patient pathway, including the supply chain, chain of custody, and clinical care delivery, we recognize the important roles of expert nurses, practice educators, and the wider multiprofessional team in sharing their knowledge and experience. Nurse education strategies should include referring nursing teams to facilitate seamless patient care throughout referral, treatment, and follow-up to optimize communication and appropriately meet patient and caregiver information needs.

Treatment plans can change rapidly; patients do not reach the point of treatment or relapse during admission. The involvement of disciplines such as palliative care and psychological therapy in the programme is key. The relationship between the

M. Kenyon (✉)
Department of Haematological Medicine, King's College Hospital, NHS Foundation Trust, London, UK
e-mail: michelle.kenyon@nhs.net

J. Murray
Haematology and Transplant Unit, The Christie NHS Foundation Trust, Manchester, UK
e-mail: j.murray10@nhs.net

R. Ellard
The Royal Marsden NHS Foundation Trust, London, UK
e-mail: rose.ellard@nhs.ne

D. Hutt
Department of Pediatric Hematology-Oncology and BMT, Edmond and Lily Safra Children's Hospital, Sheba Medical Center, Ramat Gan, Israel
e-mail: dhutt@sheba.health.gov.il

© The Author(s) 2022
N. Kröger et al. (eds.), *The EBMT/EHA CAR-T Cell Handbook*,
https://doi.org/10.1007/978-3-030-94353-0_40

referring and treating centre is critical, and an active dialogue between teams from the time of referral is imperative to optimize patient care.

Apheresis and Cell Collection

Nurses with the knowledge, skills, and expertise to perform CAR-T-specific apheresis procedures do so in many JACIE accredited centres following training and competency achievement. Apheresis booking is synchronized with the availability of manufacturing space in the pharmaceutical company, but timing is critical to maximize collection quality and minimize the risk of unsalvageable disease progression. Preprocedure work-up can include disease- and product-specific tests and screening. Technically, apheresis is similar to donor lymphocyte or mononuclear cell procedures but may be more challenging due to low lymphocyte counts following earlier treatments. The patients may be symptomatic due to the disease burden and previous therapies and can become unwell during harvest.

Cell Infusion

Thawing and cell infusion are performed in most centres by appropriately trained nurses. Frozen cells are shipped from the manufacturer, and thawing occurs at the bedside via a water bath or automated device. Specific training on defrosting and infusing the product is mandatory. Soft waste will be disposed of into a double clinical waste bag, tagged, numbered, and placed in a dedicated biohazard waste container. Sharp waste, e.g., syringes and vials, must be placed in sealed and lidded sharps container, which is tagged and labelled as biohazard waste. A disposal record should be maintained. PPE should be worn at all times of disposal. If clothing becomes contaminated, it should be changed immediately and disposed of as soft waste. If spillage occurs, the spill should be cleaned while wearing PPE and using Clinell red wipes or other virucidal products. Routine checks are performed at the bedside (patient ID, consent, prescription, vital signs, IV access). Premedication is administered, ensuring that no steroids are given. The cells are infused as per local policy and the product specification. The patient's vital signs are recorded during and following the infusion. All necessary documentation is completed. The infusion is usually uneventful, but intensive care and neurology services should be notified of the CAR-T infusion should their support be needed during the postinfusion period.

Patient Monitoring

The two most common toxicities following CAR-T infusion are cytokine release syndrome (CRS) and immune effector cell-associated neurotoxicity syndrome (ICANS).

CRS is the most common acute toxicity. Frequently reported symptoms are fever, hypoxia, and hypotension, which can mimic neutropenic sepsis. Thus, the patient must be treated for suspected infection with intravenous antibiotics and a full septic screen must be performed.

ICANS symptoms can be progressive and may include aphasia, an altered level of consciousness, impairment of cognitive skills, motor weakness, seizures, and cerebral oedema (Lee et al., 2019). Nurses should be aware of these symptoms, and familiarity with the patient's baseline condition aids in monitoring for subtle changes.

Vital signs of inpatients should be recorded at least once every 4 h to monitor for signs/symptoms of CRS. Patients may deteriorate quickly, and nurses should promptly report concerns to the medical team to ensure early recognition and treatment. The recommended monitoring and assessment tools for CRS and ICANS are the American Society of Transplant and Cellular Therapy CRS consensus grading (Table 1 in Chap. 26), immune effector cell-associated encephalopathy (ICE) tool (Table 1 in Chap. 27), and the ASTCT ICANS consensus grading (Table 2 in Chap. 27) (Lee et al., 2019). The CRS grade should be calculated if there is a deterioration in the patient's vital signs and reported to the medical team. The ICE score should be calculated at least twice daily. This tool is of particular benefit, as subtle handwriting changes can be an early sign of ICANS. If the ICE score is less than 10, the ASTCT ICANS grade (Table 3 in Chap. 27) should be calculated and the medical team notified of the change in the patient's condition. Patients require daily blood tests, including full blood count, biochemistry, CRP, and ferritin; some centres may have additional routine tests.

Toxicity Management

Treatment of symptoms is a key nursing role in the management of CAR-T toxicities. Patients with suspected CRS may require supportive measures, such as paracetamol, IV fluids, or supplemental oxygen. The first-line medicinal treatment for CRS is tocilizumab, an anti-IL6 monoclonal antibody given intravenously. Up to four doses can be given, at least 8 h apart. Second-line treatment for CRS is usually corticosteroids, although these are always used with caution due to the potential deleterious effect on CAR-T cell efficacy. However, ICANS is typically treated with corticosteroids as a first line because tocilizumab is a large molecule and does not cross the blood–brain barrier.

Discharge

Upon discharge, patients and their caregivers should have written information about potential side effects and who and how to contact an appropriate CAR-T member if they develop problems or concerns. Patients must be aware of the symptoms of CRS and serious neurological reactions and the need to report all symptoms to the CAR-T team immediately. If discharged prior to day 28, patients are required to remain within close proximity of the treatment centre until day 28. They are also advised not to drive for 8 weeks post-infusion or resolution of neurologic symptoms due to the risk of delayed neurotoxicity. Ideally, they should have a responsible adult as a caregiver for the first 3 months at home.

Long-Term Follow Up

In the CAR-T setting, the recommended minimum duration of follow-up is 15 years, with annual assessment, which fulfils the regulatory requirements and allows submission of longitudinal outcome data that can contribute to the growing evidence base. The range of assessments and late effects screening can vary between products and disease indications. Nurse awareness is necessary to support the patient with appointments, coordination of tests, communication of results, and escalation of patient concerns when raised. Early quality of life data show promising improvements (Tam et al. 2019) for some patients who achieve PR and CR. Survivorship care, supporting the patient and caregiver through the transition from treatment through recovery and beyond, is a key area for nurse development.

Paediatric Considerations

Currently, tisagenlecleucel (Kymriah™) is the only approved treatment for refractory/relapsed ALL in children and young adults up to 25 years of age. Apheresis in small children is considered safe but challenging because it has potentially more side effects than in adults due to the small body mass and unique physiology of children. Venous access in small children can be difficult and limits inlet rates and in some cases requires insertion of a leukapheresis catheter (Mahadeo et al. 2019). Children weighing 20–25 kg may require priming of the machine with packed red cells prior to the apheresis procedure. Metabolic complications due to citrate toxicity may present differently in children (Del Fante et al. 2018). Obtaining a sufficient number of harvested cells could be a limiting factor in infants and small children (Hayden et al. 2021). In the pre-apheresis consultation, the nurse should consider all of the above issues and provide age-appropriate preparation for the procedure, including descriptions of the sequence of events that will occur and accurate information on what pain and sensations to expect.

Hypotension and hypoxia are the principal determinants of the consensus grading scale, and hypotension assessment should account for age and the patient's individual baseline. Although the 10-point ICE assessment is useful for screening adults for encephalopathy, its use in children may be limited to those aged ≥12 years with sufficient cognitive ability to perform it. In children aged <12 years, the Cornell Assessment of Pediatric Delirium (CAPD) is recommended to aid in the overall grading of ICANS (Lee et al. 2019) (Table 40.1).

Table 40.1 Encephalopathy assessment for children age <12 years using the CAPD

Answer the following based on interactions with the child over the course of the shift

	Never, 4	Rarely, 3	Sometimes, 2	Often, 1	Always, 0
1. Does the child make eye contact with the caregiver?					
2. Are the child's actions purposeful?					
3. Is the child aware of his or her surroundings?					
4. Does the child communicate needs and wants?					
	Never, 0	Rarely, 1	Sometimes, 2	Often, 3	Always, 4
5. Is the child restless?					
6. Is the child inconsolable?					
7. Is the child underactive; very little movement while awake?					
8. Does it take the child a long time to respond to interactions?					

Adapted from Traube et al. 2021; reproduced with permission

After treatment, children with B-cell aplasia should receive immunoglobulin replacement to maintain IgG levels according to institutional guidelines for IgG substitution (i.e., ≥500 mg/dL) (Hayden et al. 2021).

For patients aged 1–2 years, the following serve as guidelines for the corresponding questions:

1. Holds gaze, prefers primary parent, looks at speaker.
2. Reaches and manipulates objects, tries to change position, if mobile may try to get up.
3. Prefers primary parent, upset when separated from preferred caregivers. Comforted by familiar objects (i.e., blanket or stuffed animal).
4. Uses single words or signs.
5. No sustained calm state.
6. Not soothed by usual comforting actions, e.g., singing, holding, talking, and reading.
7. Little if any play, efforts to sit up, pull up, and if mobile crawl or walk around.
8. Not following simple directions. If verbal, not engaging in simple dialogue with words or jargon.

Key Points

- Nurse education strategies should recognize the importance of the range of nursing roles at various stages in the CAR-T patient pathway and their differing education and training needs.
- Treatment plans may not always proceed as expected, and patients can experience sudden and significant changes.
- Apheresis is technically similar to donor lymphocyte or mononuclear cell procedures but may be more challenging due to low lymphocyte counts, poor physical condition or high symptom burden.
- Specific training on defrosting and infusing the product is mandatory.
- The two most common toxicities following CAR-T infusion are cytokine release syndrome (CRS) and immune effector cell-associated neurotoxicity syndrome (ICANS), for which patients are very closely monitored.
- Nurses must be trained in the use of the CRS and ICANS assessment tools, local escalation protocols, and treatment strategies.
- Specific considerations exist for paediatric patients, and these nurses must be trained accordingly.

References

Del Fante C, Seghatchian J, Perotti C. Reflections on methodical approaches to hematopoietic stem cell collection in children. Transfus Apher Sci. 2018;57(3):425–7. https://doi.org/10.1016/j.transci.2018.05.005.

Hayden PJ, Roddie C, Bader P, Basak GW, Bonig H, Bonini C, et al. Management of adults and children receiving CAR T-cell therapy: 2021 best practice recommendations of the European Society for Blood and Marrow Transplantation (EBMT) and the Joint Accreditation Committee of ISCT and EBMT (JACIE) and the European Haematology Association (EHA). Ann Oncol. 2021;S0923–7534(21):04876–6. https://doi.org/10.1016/j.annonc.2021.12.003. Online ahead of print.

Lee DW, Santomasso BD, Locke FL, Ghobadi A, Turtle CJ, Brudno JN, et al. ASTCT consensus grading for cytokine release syndrome and neurologic toxicity associated with immune effector cells. Biol Blood Marrow Transplant. 2019;25(4):625–38. https://doi.org/10.1016/j.bbmt.2018.12.758.

Mahadeo KM, Khazal SJ, Abdel-Azim H, Fitzgerald JC, Taraseviciute A, Bollard CM, et al. Management guidelines for paediatric patients receiving chimeric antigen receptor T cell therapy. Nat Rev Clin Oncol. 2019;16(1):45–63.

Schmidts A, Wehrli M, Maus MV. Toward better understanding and management of CAR-T cell-associated toxicity. Annu Rev Med. 2021;72:365–82.

Tam C, Waller E, Jaeger U, Pacaud L, Ma Q, Maziarz R. Prolonged improvement in patient reported quality of life (QoL) following tisagenlecleucel infusion in adult patients (pts) with relapsed/refractory (r/r) diffuse large B-cell lymphoma (DLBCL): 19-month follow-up (FU) of the Juliet study. BBMT. 2019;25(3):181–2.

Traube C, Gerber LM, Mauer EA, Small K, Broglie L, Chopra YR, et al. Delirium in children undergoing hematopoietic cell transplantation: a multi-institutional point prevalence study. Front Oncol. 2021;11:627726.

Role of Pharmacists

41

Margherita Galassi and Maria Estela Moreno-Martínez

The pharmacist has a key role in the management of CAR-T therapies. Selection, ordering, reception, storage, preparation of the product for infusion, and dispensing of CAR-T therapies are some of the pharmacy service responsibilities (Black 2018; Moreno-Martínez et al. 2020; Booth et al. 2020). The pharmacist requires specific training, ensuring coordination with all the professionals in the multidisciplinary team who are involved in the management of these therapies, as summarized in Table 41.1.

The pharmacist must also know which types of CARs are available and can arrive in the future. CAR-T cells are currently indicated for the treatment of B-cell acute lymphoblastic leukaemia and diffuse large B-cell lymphoma, two haematological diseases that share expression of the CD-19 antigen, but the target antigens are potentially many; therefore, the pharmacist must receive training that takes into account new future possibilities. An example of other options is the advanced phase experimentation of CAR-T cells and anti-B-cell maturation antigen (BCMA) for multiple myeloma pathologies.

CAR-T cells are just the beginning, and CAR-Technology is being applied to other immune cells:

- CAR natural killer (NK) cells: CAR-NK.
- CAR macrophages (M): CAR–M.

M. Galassi
Centrale Produzione Farmaci, Hospital Pharmacy, National Cancer Institute of Milan, Milan, Italy
e-mail: Margherita.Galassi@istitutotumori.mi.it

M. E. Moreno-Martínez (✉)
Department of Pharmacy, Hospital de la Santa Creu i Sant Pau, Barcelona, Spain
e-mail: MMorenoma@santpau.cat

N. Kröger et al. (eds.), *The EBMT/EHA CAR-T Cell Handbook*,
https://doi.org/10.1007/978-3-030-94353-0_41

Table 41.1 Pharmacist's responsibilities

Pharmacist-specific training
Selection and indication for CAR-T cell therapy • Review and approval for formulary addition • Patient eligibility criteria
Ordering: know each procedure to order the drug
Reception • Check integrity of the product, labelling, and temperature compliance • Check certificate of analysis
Storage and handling • Manage products stored at ultra-cold temperatures • Action plan if temperature deviation
Dispensing • Validate lymphodepleting chemotherapy and coordinate date of dispensing and time planned for infusion • Ensure chain of identity of cell product • Check defrosting procedure. Record the date and time of all the procedures
Administration: confirm procedure and doses of tocilizumab stock ready to use
Follow-up • Drugs permitted and contraindicated • Monitoring and management of toxicities • Ensure appropriate treatment is available
Patient and staff education

Finally, CAR-T cells may be effective against solid tumours, and the main problem related to the accessibility of the antigen can be solved in patients suffering from glioblastoma and neuroblastoma with the injection of the cells on site.

The complexity of these therapies requires the intervention of the pharmacist whose training must include implementation and management of advanced biotechnological procedures; therefore, specific skills not only in the preparation of classic chemotherapies and monoclonal antibodies but also in how to handle, store, and manage novel therapies and the specific medical devices that could be required are needed.

One of the most important pharmacist interventions is patient follow-up, intended to monitor toxicities, adverse events, and concomitant and contraindicated drugs. Cytokine release syndrome is an extremely serious event that must be monitored by a multidisciplinary team in which the pharmacist is the reference figure for the management of rescue drugs and pharmacovigilance studies.

> **Key Points**
> - The pharmacist requires specific training in the management of CAR-T therapies, ensuring coordination with all the professionals in the multidisciplinary team.
> - The pharmacist must know the types of CARs available and what will arrive quite soon.
> - New skills are needed to handle and store CARs and to follow-up with patients.

References

Black A. Pharmacy institutional readiness for marketed CAR-T therapy: checklists for pharmacy services. Version 3.0. Specialist Pharmacy Service; 2018. Available at: https://www.sps.nhs.uk/wp-content/uploads/2018/10/FINAL-Pharmacy-Institutional-Readiness-for-Marketed-CAR-TDec-2018.pdf

Booth JP, Kusoski CL, Kennerly-Shah JM. The pharmacist's role in chimeric antigen receptor T cell therapy. J Oncol Pharm Pract. 2020;26(7):1725–31.

Moreno-Martínez ME, Vinent-Genestar J, Muñoz-Sánchez C, Carreras-Soler MJ. Hospital pharmacist's roles and responsibilities with CAR-T medicines. Farm Hosp. 2020;44(1):26–31.

Educational Needs for Cell Processing Facility Personnel

42

Boris Calmels

Training on ATMP processes and procedures is systematically provided by the sponsor after site certification/accreditation.

Chain of Identity (COI) and Chain of Custody (COC) are the most crucial items to understand to ensure traceability and identification of a cellular product; for commercial ATMPs, the COI and COC are usually managed through a dedicated secure web-based platform.

In the autologous setting, cell processing staff is involved in most of the on-site ATMP stages, from collection to administration: the information flow between all protagonists must be well established to allow for timely delivery of information.

Pivotal training steps for cell processing staff:

- before apheresis: receipt of empty shipper (if apheresis is shipped after cryo-preservation) and materials.
- after apheresis completion: control of product label, sampling, cryopreservation, and/or packaging for transportation of fresh or frozen apheresis to the manufacturing site.

The responsibility for subsequent steps might be shared with or fulfilled by the hospital pharmacy, depending on local regulations.

- after manufacturing completion and prior to initiating lymphodepletion: receipt of shipper, conformity of transport temperature, frozen bag integrity, and transfer of frozen product to on-site storage.
- the day of infusion: transport of bag(s) to the thawing site, clinical ward (if bedside), or cell therapy facility (recommended) if localized near the infusion site (thawed ATMPs need to be infused asap).

B. Calmels (✉)
Cell Therapy Facility, Institut Paoli-Calmettes, Marseilles, France
e-mail: calmelsb@ipc.unicancer.fr

© The Author(s) 2022
N. Kröger et al. (eds.), *The EBMT/EHA CAR-T Cell Handbook*,
https://doi.org/10.1007/978-3-030-94353-0_42

Frozen bag handling and thawing require expertise and must be performed by experienced, i.e., cell processing staff, whenever possible: this will also relieve training of unexperienced staff, especially regarding the risks associated with liquid nitrogen exposure, and anoxia or handling of accidental bag failures.

One of the many challenges of training is to become used to the quantity and variety of forms associated with each step of the ATMP circuit; consequently, mock (training) runs organized by sponsors are pivotal for staff training.

> **Key Points**
> - Chain of Custody (COC) is crucial to ensure traceability through the multiple steps and stakeholders in the supply chain.
> - Information that flows between all protagonists must be well defined.
> - Frozen bag handling and thawing should be performed by skilled cell processing staff.

GoCART

43

Sofie R. Terwel, Jürgen Kuball, Martin Dreyling,
and Francesco Cerisoli

Cellular therapies manufactured from cells of haematopoietic origin, such as CAR-T–cell therapies, provide a revolutionary treatment for patients suffering from haematological diseases. Nonetheless, there are considerable challenges in the implementation of these therapies in this rapidly evolving field. These challenges include but are not limited to the complexity of the supply chains for these living drugs and the management of side effects, requiring centre qualification as well as additional and ongoing education of health care professionals; the long-term follow-up of patients treated with therapies with curative intent; the myriad regulatory requirements at the European Union and local level; and reimbursement of the treatments by budget-constrained authorities.

The challenges in the field of cellular therapies require cross-stakeholder collaboration, including patient representatives, health care professionals, pharmaceutical companies, health authorities, health technology assessment (HTA) bodies and reimbursement agencies, and medical organizations at both the European and national levels. For these reasons, EBMT and EHA have launched the GoCART

S. R. Terwel (✉)
EBMT GoCART, Leiden, The Netherlands
e-mail: GoCART@ebmt.org

J. Kuball
Department of Hematology, and Center for Translational Immunology, University Medical Center Utrecht, Utrecht, The Netherlands

Legal Regulatory Affairs Committee (LRAC) of EBMT, Barcelona, Spain
e-mail: j.h.e.kuball@umcutrecht.nl

M. Dreyling
Department of Medicine III, Ludwig Maximilians University Munich, Munich, Germany
e-mail: Martin.Dreyling@med.uni-muenchen.de

F. Cerisoli
EHA, The Hague, The Netherlands
e-mail: f.cerisoli@ehaweb.org

© The Author(s) 2022
N. Kröger et al. (eds.), *The EBMT/EHA CAR-T Cell Handbook*,
https://doi.org/10.1007/978-3-030-94353-0_43

221

Coalition, a multistakeholder initiative aiming to promote patient access to novel cellular therapies manufactured from cells and tissues of haematopoietic origin and to contribute to health and well-being through innovation via multistakeholder collaboration on clinical data, standards of care, education, and policy.

The aims of the GoCART coalition:

- Improve health outcomes for patients.
- Engage stakeholders and establish a sustainable European coalition in the field of cellular therapy.
- Collaborate and share data and knowledge to prevent duplication of effort and maximize resources.
- Promote harmonization of data collection, education, standards of care, regulatory approval, and reimbursement processes in Europe.
- Set up a pre- and post-marketing registry that supports regulatory decision-making and shared research purposes.
- Develop a cellular therapy education and information programme for patients and health care professionals.
- Harmonize standards of care and centre qualification.
- Advance policies that further the shared mission and vision.

The coalition is open to all stakeholders relevant to achieving its mission. Both institutional and individual members are invited to participate in work packages that implement the Coalition's mission, vision, and goals. Work package chairs are accountable to an executive committee with a balanced representation of stakeholders, and the executive committee functions as the primary decision-making body and determines the overall strategy of the coalition.

The following content work packages have been created:

1. Data harmonization
   a. Context: In Europe, clinical data from patients treated with gene and cellular therapies are reported to many registries, each built for a limited purpose, with different governance rules and specific software tools managing the data. This results in siloed data, inefficiencies, and duplication of efforts.
   b. Overall aim: Create a central EU data registry for harmonized collection of clinical data on patients treated with cellular therapies to support collaborative studies and regulatory decision-making.
2. Standards of care
   a. Context: Gene and cellular therapies are inherently complex products, and treatment administration is restricted to qualified centres. With rapid developments and pending product approvals, there is a need to develop treatment guidelines and harmonize centre qualification procedures across pharmaceutical companies, accreditation bodies, and national requirements.
   b. Overall aims: (1) To develop harmonized guidelines on patient and product management for health care professionals; (2) to reduce inspection burden and redundancies by developing and implementing consensus-driven

requirements and qualification standards for clinical teams delivering gene and cellular therapies from cells and tissues of haematopoietic origin.

3. HTA process
   a. Context: Health technology assessment bodies and reimbursement agencies need to make decisions based on the best available estimates of the properties and impact of new therapies. This is particularly challenging for gene and cellular therapies, considering that authorizations may be based on small patient groups, limited availability of (long-term) follow-up and comparator data, the high costs of the products, and the increasing number of therapies on the horizon. Although national procedures on health technology assessments and reimbursement vary considerably, there is a common need for reliable safety and effectiveness data.
   b. Overall aim: Leveraging the central registry for gene and cellular therapy as a suitable data source for health technology assessment.

4. Education
   a. Context: Gene and cellular therapies are complex products that require comprehensive and ongoing training of health care professionals as well as patients and caregivers. A plethora of training courses are already offered by MAHs as well as health organizations, which can lead to considerable overlap.
   b. Overall aim: Develop harmonized educational programmes for different groups of health care professionals and patients.

5. Policy and advocacy
   a. Context: Gene and cellular therapies are subject to EU and national regulations affecting their preparation, administration and patient access. These new therapies challenge these regulations, which were designed for more traditional pharmaceutical products, and health authorities are assessing how they will adapt.
   b. Overall aim: Represent and promote the interests of the GoCART coalition and its stakeholders in EU policy-making by engaging with EU institutions and other relevant stakeholders.

6. Scientific excellence
   a. Context: Scientific research on gene and cellular therapies has increased substantially in recent years. With real-world data becoming increasingly available, many scientific questions can be explored from different perspectives. Only by working together can we leverage enough data to conduct meaningful research. GoCART wants to maximize the use of data collected in the central registry as well as data available to other stakeholders and to facilitate further collaboration between stakeholders. While strongly protecting confidentiality, the guiding principle should be 'collect once, use often' to advance our knowledge in the field of gene and cellular therapies, support better decision-making, and drive efficiencies for all stakeholders.
   b. Overall aim: Stimulate scientific discussion across stakeholders, facilitate the setup of joint research projects, and avoid duplication of scientific efforts.

Key Points
- The GoCART cell coalition is a multistakeholder initiative in the field of cellular therapies for haematological disease.
- Stakeholders include patient representatives, health care professionals, pharmaceutical companies, health authorities, health technology assessment (HTA) bodies and reimbursement agencies, and medical organizations at both the European and national levels.
- The mission is to promote patient access to novel cellular therapies manufactured from cells and tissues of haematopoietic origin and to contribute to health and well-being through innovation via multistakeholder collaboration on clinical data, standards of care, education, and policy.
- The GoCART Coalition aims to achieve its mission through activities organized in work packages on (1) data harmonization, (2) standards of care, (3) HTA, (4) education, (5) policy and advocacy, and (6) scientific excellence.

Take a look at our webpage for the most recent information: https://thegocartcoalition.com

Patient Referral

44

John Snowden and Rafael F. Duarte

Early and efficient patient referral is a critical step in the ability of potential candidates to access CAR-T therapy. Despite improvements in centre qualification and availability, regulatory and reimbursement frameworks, and addressing the educational needs of the various members of the health care team, referring haematologists and oncologists identify major barriers to prescribing CAR-T therapy, including cumbersome logistics, high cost and toxicity, and clinical challenges, such as deterioration of the patient prior to CAR-T administration and the need for bridging chemotherapy while awaiting manufacturing (Chavarría 2021).

Pathways for referral vary between countries and regions, but generally, patients are referred to the regional CAR-T specialist multidisciplinary team (MDT) according to agreed pathways, which in turn, may be linked with national committees often necessary for additional clinical support and/or to confirm funding. These specialist MDTs confirm patient eligibility in line with the manufacturer's licence and based on diagnosis, age, fitness, disease, and treatment stage. Thereafter, the CAR-T centres will arrange to assess the patient directly (with their carers) and provide detailed information enabling the patient to understand the potential benefits, risks, and complications of treatment and to provide informed consent.

Irrespective of the treatment site, clinicians must consider the eligibility of potential patients for CAR-T cells at an early stage so that strategic decisions can be made regarding the best therapeutic pathway. Eligibility should be directly confirmed with regard to age, fitness, disease, and treatment stage. In addition, referring

J. Snowden (✉)
Department of Haematology, Sheffield Teaching Hospitals NHS Foundation Trust and University of Sheffield, Sheffield, UK
e-mail: john.snowden1@nhs.net

R. F. Duarte
Department of Hematology, Hospital Universitario Puerta de Hierro Majadahonda and Universidad Autónoma de Madrid, Madrid, Spain
e-mail: rafael.duarte@salud.madrid.org

© The Author(s) 2022
N. Kröger et al. (eds.), *The EBMT/EHA CAR-T Cell Handbook*,
https://doi.org/10.1007/978-3-030-94353-0_44

clinicians should inform their patients of the potential of using CAR-T cells in their treatment early in the pathway, especially if treatment may take place in another centre some distance from their home or base centre (Gajra et al. 2020). In addition to confirmation of eligibility and logistical arrangements with the treatment site, prompt referral and good communication are also desirable to plan the salvage protocol for bridging CAR-T therapy, particularly because defined recovery periods may be required before leukapheresis and the quality of circulating T-cells may decrease with increasing chemotherapy exposure. Sometimes patients without a high peripheral disease burden and sufficient circulating T-cells (e.g., total lymphocyte count of $>0.5 \times 10^9$/L or a peripheral blood CD3 count of >150 per µl) may be able to undergo leukapheresis for CAR-T cells before starting salvage therapy for relapse. For other patients, planning bridging therapy with the CAR-T therapy centre will be necessary. Therapies likely to significantly impair lymphocyte number and/or function should be avoided to allow successful leukapheresis for CAR-T cell therapy. Therefore, careful scheduling and prioritization of patients is required, including planning for leukapheresis, particularly given that CAR-T manufacture can take over one month. Finally, capacity planning is required for subsequent stages of care in the CAR-T centre, and later, shared care arrangements will enable continuity of care after a patient returns home (Maus and Levine 1996).

> **Key Points**
> - Prompt early patient referral from the base hospital to the treatment centre facilitates various aspects of the planning for CAR-T therapy.
> - The learning curve in the CAR-T therapy framework will also inform and facilitate the management and referral of patients for other advanced therapy medicinal products.

References

Chavarría T. Real-world regulatory issues in the implementation of advanced therapies. Multistakeholder forum at 47th EBMT annual meeting. 2021. Available at www.ebmt.org

Gajra A, Jeune-Smith Y, Kish J, Yeh T-C, Hime S, Feinberg B. Perceptions of community hematologists/oncologists on barriers to chimeric antigen receptor T-cell therapy for the treatment of diffuse large B-cell lymphoma. Immunotherapy. 2020;12(10):725–32. https://doi.org/10.2217/imt-2020-0118.

Maus MV, Levine BL. Chimeric antigen receptor T-cell therapy for the community oncologist. Oncologist. 1996;21:608–17. https://doi.org/10.1634/theoncologist.2015-0421.

Treatment Coverage and Reimbursement

45

Cornelie Haag

The conditions for reimbursement for CAR-T cell therapy are not uniform in Europe. Most European countries use a DRG system for billing hospital services, but the details vary. Nonetheless, the similarity is that expensive therapies, such as CAR-T cell therapy, are initially not included in the DRG system. Most countries possess instruments to ensure the financing of such expensive therapies outside the DRG system as separate payments. These reimbursement instruments of DRG systems are used in most countries both for short-term financing for innovative and new therapies and as long-term additional fees within the respective DRG system. Individual countries maintain different regulations, and therefore, hospitals have the responsibility to determine the specific requirements of their country before establishing CAR-T cell therapy.

One should consider that other significant costs exist in addition to the price of the actual CAR-T cell product, which has been agreed upon with the pharmaceutical industry. In addition to the usual hospitalization costs, the price of the inpatient stay for the administration of CAR-T cells can include the costs for intensive care and expensive medication, such as tocilizumab. These additional costs are generally reimbursed through the established system in each country. However, at least 2 years are required to integrate the costs of a new therapy or method into the existing DRG.

The special feature of CAR-T cell therapy is that the hospital needs to collect lymphocytes from the patient in advance through apheresis. This initial product for the production of CAR-T cells induces further costs that are usually not reimbursed.

The implementation of this new therapy in a hospital should not be underestimated. In addition to the training of staff for this new type of therapy, high demands are placed on quality management by both the pharmaceutical industry and the government. These structural costs (mostly personnel costs) for the hospital must be

C. Haag (✉)
University Hospital Carl Gustav Carus Dresden, Dresden, Germany
e-mail: Cornelie.Haag@uniklinikum-dresden.de

© The Author(s) 2022
N. Kröger et al. (eds.), *The EBMT/EHA CAR-T Cell Handbook*,
https://doi.org/10.1007/978-3-030-94353-0_45

agreed upon separately with health insurance companies or the government, depending on the state-dependent reimbursement system.

A single hospital has a minor impact on the pricing of a CAR-T cell product; this is usually done by negotiation between pharmaceutical companies and government agencies.

In addition to the reimbursement of the CAR-T cell product at the price set by these negotiations, the additional costs of this therapy are reimbursed differently, particularly within Germany. Efforts are being made to centralize these negotiations, but the success of such a centralized negotiation depends on the structures and organization of the numerous health insurance companies in Germany.

In Germany, the individual hospital then becomes responsible for the specific reimbursement of costs for each individual patient. In the case of extremely high costs, advanced agreements are usually made between the health insurance and the hospital.

Before initiating CAR-T cell therapy, every doctor or hospital should be aware of the different regulations in each country to avoid not receiving reimbursement for this expensive therapy.

Key Points
- Different rules in different countries.
- Additional costs aside from the cost of the CAR-T cell product.

The Value of CAR-T-cell Immunotherapy in Cancer

Mohamed Abou-el-Enein and Jordan Gauthier

The development of genetically modified chimeric antigen receptor (CAR) T-cells to target cancer by conferring tumour antigen recognition has tremendously improved the fight against the disease and broadened treatment options for haematological malignancies (Elsallab et al. 2020b). However, in contrast to conventional drugs that patients can easily access, the implementation of CAR-T-cell therapy in routine clinical practice poses significant challenges. Access to CAR-T-cell products is currently limited to specific certified centres meeting the requirements set up by manufacturers and regulatory agencies. There are also issues regarding insurance coverage, reimbursement, affordability, and pricing, which have critical impacts on broadening patient access to these novel therapies (Abou-El-Enein et al. 2016a, b). Current list pricing ranges between \$373,000 and \$475,000 per one-time infusion for the five CAR-T-cell therapies currently approved by the FDA (tisagenlecleucel, Kymriah®; axicabtagene ciloleucel, Yescarta®; brexucabtagene autoleucel, Tecartus®; lisocabtagene maraleucel, Breyanzi®; idecabtagene vicleucel, Abecma®). In addition to the cost of the CAR-T-cell product, patient preparation (leukapheresis and/or lymphodepletion), product infusion, pre- and post-infusion patient management, and monitoring for side effects (Wagner et al. 2021) significantly add to the final price tag. There are calls for restructuring the current payment and

M. Abou-el-Enein (✉)
Division of Medical Oncology, Department of Medicine, and Department of Stem Cell Biology and Regenerative Medicine, Keck School of Medicine, University of Southern California, Los Angeles, CA, USA

Joint USC/CHLA Cell Therapy Program, University of Southern California, and Children Hospital, Los Angeles, CA, USA
e-mail: abouelenein@med.usc.edu

J. Gauthier
Clinical Research Division, Fred Hutchinson Cancer Research Center, Seattle, WA, USA

Division of Medical Oncology, University of Washington, Seattle, WA, USA
e-mail: jgauthier@fredhutch.org

© The Author(s) 2022
N. Kröger et al. (eds.), *The EBMT/EHA CAR-T Cell Handbook*,
https://doi.org/10.1007/978-3-030-94353-0_46

reimbursement models to allow better access to CAR-T-cell therapies (Abou-El-Enein et al. 2014). However, this would only be possible after examining the strength of clinical evidence generated during product development (Abou-El-Enein and Hey 2019; Elsallab et al. 2020a) and, most importantly, by determining the value of CAR-T-cell therapy.

Efficacy does not automatically entail value. Quality-adjusted life years (QALYs) per dollar spent reflect a well-accepted measure of cost-effectiveness to assess value. QALYs enable evaluation of the impact of a certain therapy on the entire lifespan of a patient (quantity of life) and on health-related quality of life (HRQoL), reflecting a main parameter of treatment outcomes (Whitehead and Ali 2010). As composite estimates of mortality and morbidity, QALYs are conventionally calculated by accumulating life years attained from a utility value specific to certain health states. Preference elicitation studies in patients with a certain medical condition, such as in clinical trial scenarios, or in the general population serve as the basis to derive this utility value (Prieto and Sacristán 2003; Whitehead and Ali 2010; Sanders et al. 2016; Fiorenza et al. 2020).

Various models have been utilized to assess the cost-effectiveness of CAR-T-cell therapy. With respect to Kymriah® and Yescarta®, Lin et al. used a decision analytic Markov model and data from multicentre single-arm trials from a US health payer perspective for patients with relapsed or refractory (r/r) adult large B-cell lymphoma. CAR-T-cell therapies were compared to salvage chemotherapy and stem cell transplantation by incorporating certain assumptions regarding long-term effectiveness in the model. Yescarta® was shown to prolong life expectancy by 8.2 years at $129,000/QALY gained (95% uncertainty interval, $90,000 to $219,000) when assuming a 40% 5-year progression-free survival (PFS). Kymriah® led to an increase of 4.6 years at $168,000/QALY gained (95% uncertainty interval, $105,000 to $414,000/QALY) when assuming a 35% 5-year PFS (Lin et al. 2019). The study indicated that lowering the list price of Yescarta® and Kymriah® to $250,000 and $200,000 in the US, respectively, or implementing payment only for an initial complete response (at current prices) would enable both CAR-T-cell therapies to cost less than $150,000/QALY even at the more conservative assumption of a 25% 5-year PFS (Lin et al. 2019). Using data of paediatric patients with r/r B-cell ALL, Sarkar et al. built a microsimulation model to measure the incremental cost-effectiveness ratio (ICER) (Sanders et al. 2016) comparing CAR-T-cell therapy to standard of care, considering ICERs below a threshold of $100,000 per QALY as cost-effective (Sarkar et al. 2019). Assuming a 76% 1-year survival, they demonstrated an increase in overall cost by $528,200 with improved effectiveness by 8.18 QALYs, leading to an ICER of $64,600/QALY. However, if the assumption was modified to 57.8% 1-year survival, CAR-T-cell therapy in paediatric B-ALL patients was no longer cost-effective. While probabilistic sensitivity analysis showed CAR-T-cell therapy to be cost-effective in approximately 95% of iterations at a level of willingness to pay $100,000/QALY (Sarkar et al. 2019), assumptions made regarding long-term outcomes in both models need to be confirmed by real-world data with longer follow-up duration to enable robust validation of study outcomes.

When discussing value-based considerations, social value gained by CAR-T-cell therapy in the long term should also be taken into account. Offering a cure to paediatric cancer patients would enable them to lead a more productive life (Fiorenza et al. 2020). Moreover, successful milestones reached with respect to patenting (Jürgens and Clarke 2019) and regulatory and clinical success (Elsallab et al. 2020b) will increase public recognition, financial support, and advancements in the entire cellular therapy field. A recent study applied an economic framework to measure the social value of CAR-T-cell therapy as a sum of consumer surplus and profit for the manufacturing company (Thornton Snider et al. 2019). Consumer surplus reflected the difference between the added value of health gains achieved by the therapy and its incremental cost, accounting also for indirect costs and patient benefits. The gained social value was determined to be as much as $6.5 billion and $34.8 billion for paediatric ALL and DLBCL, respectively, with a net social value gain of $952,991 per child treated for B-ALL, even after including costs for production and treatment. However, they also showed a critical effect of treatment delays that negatively affect the social value generated by CAR-T-cell therapy, with a 1, 2, or 6 month treatment delay leading to a 9.8%, 36.2%, and 67.3% loss of social value, respectively, for paediatric ALL patients and a 4.2%, 11.5%, and 46.0% loss of social value, respectively, for patients with DLBCL (Thornton Snider et al. 2019). Thus, timely patient access is a key factor in the level of value achieved. Other key parameters to optimize the value of CAR-T-cell therapies rely on improving response rates, minimizing the risk of relapse and lowering the costs of toxicity management (Fiorenza et al. 2020).

Although CAR-T-cell therapy is undoubtedly transforming the therapeutic landscape for cancer patients, significant economic challenges ought to be addressed to allow broader and fairer access to these new therapies. Since most cost-effectiveness models are highly assumption-sensitive, a longer follow-up duration is warranted to better assess the value of CAR-T-cell therapies compared to alternative approaches.

Key Points
- CAR-T-cells have emerged as an important therapeutic approach for many cancer patients; however, issues regarding insurance coverage, reimbursement, affordability and pricing impact access to these novel therapies.
- Short-term clinical data have demonstrated the potential of CAR-T-cells to become a cost-effective approach for cancer patients, but availability of long-term clinical outcomes will be required to achieve this goal.
- The value of such a novel therapeutic modality should also be evaluated within the social gains of cancer patients resuming normal and productive lifestyles. However, these gains are dramatically influenced by delays in receiving the treatments.

References

Abou-El-Enein M, Hey SP. Cell and gene therapy trials: are we facing an "evidence crisis"? EClinicalMedicine. 2019;7:13–4. https://doi.org/10.1016/j.eclinm.2019.01.015.

Abou-El-Enein M, Bauer G, Reinke P. The business case for cell and gene therapies. Nat Biotechnol. 2014;32(12):1192–3. https://doi.org/10.1038/nbt.3084.

Abou-El-Enein M, Elsanhoury A, Reinke P. Overcoming challenges facing advanced therapies in the EU market. Cell Stem Cell. 2016a;12:293–7. https://doi.org/10.1016/j.stem.2016.08.012.

Abou-El-Enein M, et al. Putting a price tag on novel autologous cellular therapies. Cytotherapy. 2016b;18(8):1056–61. https://doi.org/10.1016/j.jcyt.2016.05.005.

Elsallab M, Bravery CA, et al. Mitigating deficiencies in evidence during regulatory assessments of advanced therapies: a comparative study with other biologicals. Mol Ther. 2020a;18:269–79. https://doi.org/10.1016/j.omtm.2020.05.035.

Elsallab M, Levine BL, et al. CAR-T-cell product performance in haematological malignancies before and after marketing authorisation. In: The lancet oncology. Amsterdam: Elsevier; 2020b. p. 104–16. https://doi.org/10.1016/S1470-2045(19)30729-6.

Fiorenza S, et al. Value and affordability of CAR-T-cell therapy in the United States. Bone Marrow Transplant. 2020;55(9):1706–15. https://doi.org/10.1038/s41409-020-0956-8.

Jürgens B, Clarke NS. Evolution of CAR-T -cell immunotherapy in terms of patenting activity. Nat Biotechnol. 2019;37(4):370–5. https://doi.org/10.1038/s41587-019-0083-5.

Lin JK, et al. Cost effectiveness of chimeric antigen receptor T-Cell therapy in multiply relapsed or refractory adult large B-cell lymphoma. J Clin Oncol. 2019;37(24):2105–19. https://doi.org/10.1200/JCO.18.02079.

Prieto L, Sacristán JA. Problems and solutions in calculating quality-adjusted life years (QALYs). Health Qual Life Outcomes. 2003;1:80. https://doi.org/10.1186/1477-7525-1-80.

Sanders GD, et al. Recommendations for conduct, methodological practices, and reporting of cost-effectiveness analyses. JAMA. 2016;316(10):1093. https://doi.org/10.1001/jama.2016.12195.

Sarkar RR, et al. Cost-effectiveness of chimeric antigen receptor T-cell therapy in pediatric relapsed/refractory B-cell acute lymphoblastic leukemia. J Natl Cancer Inst. 2019;111(7):719–26. https://doi.org/10.1093/jnci/djy193.

Thornton Snider J, et al. The potential impact of CAR-T-cell treatment delays on society. Am J Manag Care. 2019;25(8):379–86.

Wagner DL, et al. Immunogenicity of CAR-T cells in cancer therapy. Nat Rev Clin Oncol. 2021. https://doi.org/10.1038/s41571-021-00476-2.

Whitehead SJ, Ali S. Health outcomes in economic evaluation: the QALY and utilities. Br Med Bull. 2010;96(1):5–21. https://doi.org/10.1093/bmb/ldq033.

What do Patients Want? The Importance of Patient-reported Outcomes

Hélène Schoemans, Natacha Bolaños, and Lorna Warwick

Understanding of what it means for patients to receive CAR-T therapy remains insufficient due to the small number of studies with a quality of life (QOL) focus, selection bias of respondents, high risk of attrition due to disease relapse, and limited length of follow-up. CAR-T therapy is often presented as a last option for patients with advanced disease. The primary aim of the treatment is patient survival and hopefully disease elimination. However, understanding other aspects of health, such as functional status, cognitive function, psychosocial concerns, and other health-related (QOL) issues, is key to appreciating the full impact of such therapies at both the individual and societal levels.

Such information can only be accessed by asking patients and caregivers directly, without going through the filter of a third party, using either patient-reported outcome measures and/or qualitative methods, such as interviews or focus groups. This approach is supported by the cell therapy community, but evidence remains limited (Chakraborty et al. 2019; Shalabi et al. 2021).

Side effects, such as CRS, neurotoxicity, and B-cell aplasia, are well documented. Importantly, many patients report other concerns that impact their well-being and require appropriate support from their health care team (Bamigbola et al. 2021).

H. Schoemans (✉)
Department of Hematology, University Hospitals Leuven, Leuven, Belgium

Department of Public Health and Primary Care, ACCENT VV, Katholieke Universiteit Leuven - University of Leuven, Leuven, Belgium
e-mail: helene.schoemans@uzleuven.be

N. Bolaños
Lymphoma Coalition, Madrid, Spain
e-mail: natachab@lymphomacoalition.org

L. Warwick
Lymphoma Coalition, Management, Mississauga, ON, Canada
e-mail: lorna@lymphomacoalition.org

© The Author(s) 2022
N. Kröger et al. (eds.), *The EBMT/EHA CAR-T Cell Handbook*,
https://doi.org/10.1007/978-3-030-94353-0_47

Hoogland and colleagues recently showed that over half of adult CAR-T recipients complained of moderate to severe fatigue (84%), decreased appetite (73%), dry mouth (61%), and insomnia (55%) in the first 100 days following therapy, with a symptom peak seen after approximately two weeks (Hoogland et al. 2021). Compared to baseline, physical functioning significantly improved, with decreased pain, fatigue, and depression, but anxiety increased (Hoogland et al. 2021). In a follow-up study up to 1-year post-CAR-T cell infusion, approximately one-third of patients presented lasting moderate to severe fatigue and insomnia, and 20% had decreased memory compared to baseline (Barata et al. 2021). In contrast, in children and adolescents (3–21 years) who had undergone CAR-T therapy for acute leukaemia, a steady significant improvement in QOL compared to baseline was seen from 3 months post-treatment in all domains examined (Laetsch et al. 2019).

Mental health is a long-term issue, considering that up to 20% of 1 to 5-year adult survivors reported clinically meaningful depression or anxiety and over one-third experienced cognitive difficulties (Ruark et al. 2020). Marziaz and colleagues also showed meaningful improvement in QOL up to month 18 in all domains, except for mental health (Maziarz et al. 2020). Of note, there have been no significant associations identified between the severity of CRS or ICANS and long-term quality of life to date.

Little is known about patient priorities and needs after CAR-T therapy, but the current literature underscores the importance of appropriate information. By interviewing patients, Matthews et al. found that most felt unprepared for the emotional aspects of CAR-T therapy nor were they prepared for the intensity of the toxicities (Matthews et al. 2019). The importance of addressing issues, such as clear information on the treatment trajectory (Bamigbola et al. 2021), financial toxicity, and the importance of family members and other caregivers, has also been described (Foster et al. 2020).

Future studies are needed to broaden the understanding of CAR-T cell therapy survivorship to identify the themes most important to patients, potentially including themes identified in other cell therapy recipients, such as impact on informal caregivers, return to school/work, financial issues, and access to care (Burns et al. 2018). Outcome evaluation in large groups of patients with extended longitudinal follow-up is particularly important to identify predictors of QOL, specifically of mental health and cognitive function, so patients undergoing CAR-T therapy can be better informed and supported.

Key Points
- Symptom burden generally decreases over time, starting from 3 months post CAR-T therapy.
- Mental health and cognitive function remain a concern in long-term survivors.
- Currently, there is no indication of an association between CRS or ICANs and long-term QOL.
- Patient priorities, expectations, and needs regarding CAR-T cell therapy urgently need to be assessed.

References

Bamigbola O, Dren N, Warwick L. Cross-sectional study of the side-effects profile and patient-doctor communication about side effects in patients with lymphoma treated with CAR-T therapy. Poster presented at: 3rd European CAR-T -cell Meeting 2021, Virtual, 2021.

Barata A, Hoogland AI, Hyland K, Kommalapati A, Irizarry-Arroyo N, Rodriguez Y, et al. Patient-reported toxicities in axicabtagene ciloleucel recipients: 1-year follow-up. Transplant Cell Ther. 2021;27(3):375.

Burns LJ, Abbetti B, Arnold SD, Bender J, Doughtie S, El-Jawahiri A, et al. Engaging patients in setting a patient-centered outcomes research agenda in hematopoietic cell transplantation. Biol Blood Marrow Transplant. 2018;24(6):1111–8.

Chakraborty R, Sidana S, Shah GL, Scordo M, Hamilton BK, Majhail NS. Patient-reported outcomes with chimeric antigen receptor T cell therapy: challenges and opportunities. Biol Blood Marrow Transplant. 2019;25(5):155–62.

Foster M, Fergusson DA, Hawrysh T, Presseau J, Kekre N, Schwartz S, et al. Partnering with patients to get better outcomes with chimeric antigen receptor T-cell therapy: towards engagement of patients in early phase trials. Res Involve Engage. 2020;6:61.

Hoogland AI, Jayani RV, Collier A, Irizarry-Arroyo N, Rodriguez Y, Jain MD, et al. Acute patient-reported outcomes in B-cell malignancies treated with axicabtagene ciloleucel. Cancer Med. 2021;10(6):1936–43.

Laetsch TW, Myers GD, Baruchel A, Dietz AC, Pulsipher MA, Bittencourt H, et al. Patient-reported quality of life after tisagenlecleucel infusion in children and young adults with relapsed or refractory B-cell acute lymphoblastic leukaemia: a global, single-arm, phase 2 trial. Lancet. 2019;20(12):1710–8.

Matthews A, Sidana S, Seymour L, Pick N, Pringnitz J, Argue D, et al. QIM19-136: developing an Ideal CAR-T cell therapy patient experience through human-centered design and innovation. J Natl Compr Cancer Netw. 2019;17:3–5.

Maziarz RT, Waller EK, Jaeger U, Fleury I, McGuirk J, Holte H, et al. Patient-reported long-term quality of life after tisagenlecleucel in relapsed/refractory diffuse large B-cell lymphoma. Blood Adv. 2020;4(4):629–37.

Ruark J, Mullane E, Cleary N, Cordeiro A, Bezerra ED, Wu V, et al. Patient-reported neuropsychiatric outcomes of long-term survivors after chimeric antigen receptor T cell therapy. Biol Blood Marrow Transplant. 2020;26(1):34–43.

Shalabi H, Gust J, Taraseviciute A, Wolters PL, Leahy AB, Sandi C, et al. Beyond the storm - subacute toxicities and late effects in children receiving CAR-T cells. Clin Oncol. 2021;18(6):363–78.